MAKING
THE SYSTEM <u>WORK</u>
FOR YOUR CHILD
WITH ADHD

MAKING THE SYSTEM WORK FOR YOUR CHILD

A Guilford Series
Peter S. Jensen, *Series Editor*

Making the System Work for Your Child with ADHD
Peter S. Jensen

Forthcoming

Making the System Work for Your Child with Autism
Bryna Siegel

MAKING
THE SYSTEM <u>WORK</u>
FOR YOUR CHILD
WITH ADHD

Peter S. Jensen

THE GUILFORD PRESS
New York   London

Library of Congress Cataloging-in-Publication Data

Jensen, Peter S.
   Making the system work for your child with ADHD / Peter Jensen.
        p.   cm.
   Includes index.
   ISBN 1-57230-870-2 (pbk.) — ISBN 1-59385-027-1 (hardcover)
   1. Attention-deficit hyperactivity disorder—Popular works.
2. Attention-deficit hyperactivity disorder—Patients—Care—Popular works.   3. Parenting—Popular works.   I. Title.
   RJ506.H9J46 2004
   618.92′8589—dc22

                                                          2004005761

CONTENTS

Appendices

PREFACE

"What has made all the difference for me is learning what other parents know and knowing that I am not alone. It's too hard to try to do this all on your own."

"In my opinion, the only way to make things change is to become more involved and not just trust everything the professionals tell you."

"Trust the voice inside that is uncomfortable facing the daily challenges of ADHD and take it on, full force. The rewards are tremendous."

This book is for those who want to become experts in obtaining the best possible care for a child with attention-deficit/hyperactivity disorder (ADHD). Although I use the term *parent* throughout, I hope you'll know I'm speaking to you too, if you are an adult who finds yourself to be the primary caregiver of, and responsible for getting help for, a child with ADHD—whether you're a grandparent, a foster parent, an aunt, an older sibling, or anyone else.

Why Is This Book Needed?

In my view, ADHD is a chronic problem usually covering all of a child's growing-up years (not to mention his or her adulthood in most instances). As a result, you, like your affected youngster, are going to be dealing with the consequences of his or her ADHD for a long time, and if you are to succeed over the long haul, you will *need* to become an effective advocate for your child. In effect, then, this book is an advanced course in dealing with your child's ADHD, and it is intended to complement (rather than replace) the various comprehensive handbooks for ADHD (such as Russell Barkley's *Taking Charge of ADHD*). You can use this book alongside such other more basic books, just when you are learning more about ADHD and its management itself, or you can use it later, when you have run into the inevitable brick walls in finding the best treatment, creating the best learning environment, and/or constructing the most helpful overall program for your child.

As one parent put it, "It would have been a tremendous asset to us if someone had written a resource book pooling parents' suggestions and ideas, thereby giving us different avenues of approach to the question 'OK, now that someone suspects our child has ADHD, whom should we see? What do we do first?' " This sentiment is in fact echoed by many parents who have a child with ADHD, because tackling all of the challenges is so much more complex than just dispensing a pill or taking your child to the doctor or a therapist on a regular basis. The harsh realities of managing a chronic condition such as ADHD stretch most parents and families well beyond what they would have initially anticipated, as obstacle after obstacle arises to thwart their attempts to "fix" the problem. I go into these inevitable obstacles in more depth in Chapter 1. For now, the fact that they are equal-opportunity hurdles means that *we all need help*. I say "we," because I also have a youngster with ADHD, as well as four other children. My son with ADHD is now in his young adult years, so I can say "I've been there." But as you will learn throughout this book, I am still "there": The challenges I face have changed greatly since he was a youngster, but they don't necessarily go away.

What Is at Stake?

I often ask experienced parents who have a youngster with ADHD, particularly those who have become passionate advocates for improving the system for all children with ADHD, "Looking back now, how many years did you lose while learning how to make things work for your child?" Almost invariably, the answer is *between four and seven years*. Think of it: four or more years of your child's development (and your daily struggles) lost trying to "get it right" before you finally learn how to get your child the best care possible!

But don't despair if you've been slugging it out in the trenches for several years already and feel like you've been running in place (or even backward). As a parent or caregiver of a youngster with ADHD, you can use this book at any point along the way in the ADHD diagnosis, treatment, and long-term care of your child. Even if you've been struggling for years with your child/adolescent with ADHD, it is important to realize that it's not too late. You and your child can benefit at any point along the way by applying the concepts and principles in this book. Your child continues to develop, and you can have an impact at any point in working to improve the care and assistance that he or she receives in school, medical, and home settings. What's at stake at this point and as you look forward? Your child's current happiness and chances for future success, your family's tranquility, and possibly even some increased measure of sanity for you!

Who Needs This Book?

Well, just about anyone who wants to get the most out of a child's school, healthcare, and other supportive resources, as well as any parent or caretaker who wishes to learn how to make those resources become available by learning to work the ropes of the system and negotiate what is needed for the child, the family, and themselves. Perhaps your child has just been diagnosed and treatment only started recently. Or perhaps you have reached a later point, when you realize there's no easy way out and there are no magic bullets—that the relief of getting a correct diagnosis is not the end but the beginning of your work on your child's behalf. Or maybe you're a parent who has been out there for some time—and you've become completely frustrated and need some help in negotiating the system. Or perhaps you're simply the parent who wants the best information available: You already know how to be assertive but appreciate having lots of practical resources gathered together in one book. Regardless of where you are on this personal pilgrimage, my goal in this book is to help you become savvy in all the areas in which you need to advocate for your child: getting your money's worth from the insurance system; getting the most out of overworked, underfunded educational systems; making effective use of fleeting time with doctors and therapists; turning the teacher into an ally; and refitting household systems so that a child's ADHD doesn't excessively affect siblings and other family members.

Not all parents need the same amount of help to become savvy in all areas, however. Therefore, this book offers a range of approaches for getting what your child needs under varying circumstances, from collaborative approaches to establish an alliance with school or medical professionals at the start, to more assertive and creative approaches that may be necessary when the system isn't working as it should.

Throughout this book, I attempt to help you stay in touch with the reality that resources may be limited, helping professionals may be overwhelmed, and you may not get everything that you want or need. But by becoming experts in the system, as parents, we will stand the best chance of getting what our children need.

How Should I Use the Book?

Because my goal is to help you become an effective case manager for your child with ADHD, throughout this book you will find general tips on clear, assertive, and productive communication with mental healthcare, education, and other providers, as well as problem-solving tips from those expert parents who have gone through the process of managing their child's ADHD care. Practical tools, such as model dialogues, sample letters (to school boards, from lawyers, etc.), medication logs and other recording devices, and assertiveness and other exercises, are included in this book.

Practicality, problem solving, and putting wisdom to work are the book's repeated focus. In each chapter you will find discussions of at least three or four challenges or things to do that you couldn't or didn't do before, along with tips on how best to overcome these obstacles. If you're wrestling with any of the following questions, you'll find carefully considered answers not only from my professional experience but also from parents whose combined expertise adds up to a mountain of inventive ideas.

- What do I do when behavior therapies that sound great on paper or in the therapist's office don't work at home?
- How do I deal with an imperious doctor?
- How do I get the doctor, therapist, and teacher to collaborate with me in my child's care?
- How can I get the best medical care for my child when my insurance won't cover it?
- How can I tell when a second or third opinion is warranted?
- How do I exercise my child's legal rights when things are going haywire at school?
- How do I make my child feel "normal" when outsiders are labeling him?
- What's the best way to erase stigma and enlighten others when they are blaming me or my child for ADHD?
- How do I hold my family and my household—and myself—together while we're expending so much time and effort on managing ADHD?

Many parents who've preceded you have struggled to find answers to the same questions, and wherever possible, I tell you what they came up with—as well as their thoughts and emotions along the way—in their own words. In fact, in the preparation of this book, over eighty parents have offered specific suggestions and advice concerning the most important things they learned in working with their children and with the system, knowing that this information would reach you throughout these pages. Please note that I have protected their identities by changing various specific details—name, age, gender, and so forth. In some instances I have also edited their quotes for clarity, but the language and advice is theirs. I am most grateful to these parents, as well as to CHADD, the organization that put me in touch with these parents. CHADD (Children and Adults with Attention-Deficit/Hyperactivity Disorder), the leading parent self-help organization devoted to helping others tackle the problems of raising a child with ADHD, has greatly facilitated our shared effort through their marvelous president, Evelyn Greene, who contacted and encouraged members to contribute their advice.

Through these parents' voices, and with my own experience as a parent of a child with ADHD and as a physician, I help you systematically identify, organize, and tackle the problems you have encountered and are likely still to encounter in managing your child's ADHD. Chapter by chapter, I systematically take you through a planning/problem-solving process, helping you prioritize the various challenges you are facing, then offer guidance on how to put your plans into place. While many parts of the book are couched in these parents' own words, I bear full responsibility for the final words in my role as the book's author.

This book is divided into two parts. Part I provides general information on advocacy for ADHD. With the fundamental tools, skills, and information in this section, anyone can become an effective case manager for a child with ADHD. Part II addresses each setting in which we as parents need to advocate for our children—healthcare, education, home, and the outside world—and tells you what you should expect and how to get it when it is not happening. Straightforward factual information on ADHD is delivered in a concise fashion and limited largely to what is needed in getting the best care possible for your child. Discussion of the nature of ADHD, its course, and the range of severity is succinct and includes liberal references to other sources. So if you've already digested the factual information in the comprehensive handbooks, you won't have to sift through it again. But if not, you'll find enough such information in the following pages to let you determine whether there are areas you want to investigate more fully elsewhere.

As a physician and child psychiatrist, I have had over twenty years' experience in diagnosing and treating ADHD. I have also had the privilege of working for ten years at the National Institute of Mental Health (NIMH), where I had oversight for the nation's ADHD research programs, as well as all other areas of federally funded research on treatments of childhood mental health problems. I have since directed the Center for the Advancement of Children's Mental Health at Columbia University. Yet despite all this "professional" experience, I have been awed by the extraordinary and often superior help that I and other parents have received through the process of parents sharing their insights and accumulated wisdom. In making this wisdom more widely available by writing this book, I believe, trust, and hope that I will do parents and families a greater service than I have ever been able to do in working with families one by one in my clinical practice. In fact, from here on out, I will make it required reading!

"I beat my head against the wall for the first few years, trying to make things work," recalled one mother of a boy with ADHD. "It was a difficult time for me. So one of the reasons I got so involved is to help other parents learn what I learned. They shouldn't have to make the same mistakes I made or lose the same time I lost."

Amen.

Part I

TAKING CHARGE OF GETTING HELP FOR YOUR CHILD

One

NOWHERE TO TURN?

Why It's So Hard to Get the Help Your Child Deserves and What You Can Do about It

"The doctor means well, but his advice just isn't practical."

"The school says it is 'not their problem' because ADHD is not a school's responsibility but a medical problem."

"My husband thinks the 'real problem' with our child is that I am a pushover and 'just not firm enough.' "

"I never would have known how much my daughter could have done on long-acting medications, because my insurance company would not pay for them."

The fact that you're reading this book probably means you've run into some of the same obstacles as these parents. Despite repeated efforts and a firm commitment to helping your youngster with ADHD, "the system" just seems to stand in your way. Maybe it's the insurance company that won't cover the latest medication even though it's the only one that really seems to help your child concentrate at school. Or it could be your local school system, which just doesn't have enough funds to give your child extra help while letting him remain in a regular classroom, where you're sure he'll thrive—if only he could be allowed extra time for tests and be offered methods to help him stay on task. Perhaps "the system" is your own family—a spouse who "doesn't believe in ADHD," as one mother reported, relatives who shun your admittedly disruptive child and therefore your entire family unit, or siblings who are falling apart from the conflict and neglect they are suffering because the kid with ADHD needs so much time from you.

Far too often, the systems in place to help children with chronic illnesses like ADHD fall short, largely because the unique problems of an individual child require costly, time-consuming attention and the number of individual kids needing such care simply exceeds the capacity of the available resources. But sometimes the system *can* work for your child, if you know how to push the right buttons and pull the right levers. The trouble is, by the time you've piled up what feels like a lifetime of frustration over the system's shortcomings, you may have very little sense of what's gone wrong, much less what to do about it.

Most likely, you have already read other books on the topic of ADHD, you have consulted with your child's doctor, and perhaps you even have sought the advice of a professional counselor or therapist, such as a child psychologist or psychiatrist. Almost certainly, you have had repeated discussions with your child's teachers, and you may also have sought advice from family members and friends. So, given all the effort you have put into getting your child help, why are things still so difficult?

The short answer is that the task before you is one of the toughest any parent— and person—ever faces. As a parent of a child with ADHD, I can personally attest to a lot of trial-and-error, hit-and-miss attempts to do the right thing, only to realize later that I made yet another mistake . . . despite undergraduate training in psychology, four years of medical school, and extensive training in child, adolescent, and adult psychiatry! Creating a good life and crafting a promising future for a child with ADHD is incredibly complicated. Lest you've gotten so down on yourself for "failing" that you've forgotten what you're trying to accomplish, let me remind you how high the bar has been set for you: You have to convince an underfunded school system that may be understaffed with undertrained educators to learn and use new classroom and homework systems to ensure that your child has the same chance to learn as the dozens of other children under its tutelage. You have to work with a doctor pressured by managed care to treat patients faster and more cheaply in finding medication that will calm your child down and help him concentrate, without keeping him up at night or causing other intolerable side effects. You may very well have to negotiate with your insurance company with the skill of an experienced arbitrator to get coverage for therapy, medications, and even visits to the prescribing physician. You and your child's other parent have to set aside philosophical differences and marital conflicts to form a united front to help your son or daughter with ADHD. And you have to take on these time-consuming, exhausting tasks without neglecting your other kids, harming your own health, or going broke.

Not so short an answer after all, is it? Now for the long answer.

Why Medical Facts Are Not Enough

What has often surprised me is that while my training has definitely been helpful, it is my experiences *as a parent* (including my many mistakes) that have been most valuable in assisting parents to develop workable solutions for their child with ADHD. In fact, my experiences as a parent tend to keep me honest.

I am often aware that the simple, typical medical advice I dispense in the comfortable surroundings of my office isn't nearly enough to send a parent off knowing exactly what to do at home. The difference between what I can read in any medical textbook and what works in the "real world" lies in the particulars of adapting the advice to the given circumstances of that child and family, and in debugging the tools and techniques to be applied to the many problems that get in the way.

On a Personal Note . . .

To show you what I mean, let me give you one of my own trial-and-error experiences. As you might expect for a child psychiatrist, I spent no small amount of time in graduate and postgraduate training learning how to apply behavior therapy, a special form of treatment that relies on so-called rewards and consequences—point systems and the like—to help a child with behavioral problems such as ADHD, oppositionality, and aggression. Just in time, too, since my own son (and his parents) was dealing with ADHD-related behavior problems. So being now well trained in these methods, I began to put them to work and was getting some early, promising changes in my son's behavior. But things hit a snag after a few months, when the point program I had put into place seemed to be backfiring. To me this was a mystery not satisfactorily addressed during my training. Fortunately, my son was there to offer an explanation: "Dad, when you give me a 'consequence' and 'behavior therapy' me, it only makes me want to be badder!"

What now? Should I abandon the approach that seemed to be backfiring? Or was there some way I could modify it? Or perhaps try a few more father–son heart-to-heart talks? Turn the problem over to his mother? Or was a medication change called for? Well, in this case, discretion was the better part of valor, and I backed off. Instead I worked on strengthening the father–son relationship and on my own emotional responses to his behavior problems. I'll fill in the details in Chapter 7 of this book, where you'll find ideas for debugging various other treatment and parenting situations. My point right now is that for a condition such as ADHD, medical facts, treatments, and techniques are rarely complete solutions in and of themselves. Most often, they are only part of a long-range, big-picture strategy that must be modified, adapted, and changed in response to the daily–weekly–monthly issues and obstacles that interfere with the straight-line movement toward a goal.

Think of yourself as the skipper of a sailing vessel. At the beginning of a voyage, your craft should at minimum be outfitted with sails, a rudder, a compass and map, a radio, a knowledgeable skipper, other crew members, and adequate provisions. Even with all of these ingredients on board, and despite the fact that you, the skipper, charted an initially appropriate course at the outset, any significant change in weather is likely to dictate a change in plans, not just to adapt to the prevailing winds and adjust course, but even to make more drastic changes, such as weighing anchor at a temporary safe harbor, returning to port, or radioing the Coast Guard for help.

On your journey to getting your child the best possible care for ADHD, you may run into similar snags. You may devise a good school program for your child, but what if the teacher doesn't want to "play along"? What if the doctor doesn't seem to be up on the latest medication approaches? Or your spouse thinks the "real problem" is that you are not "firm enough"? Or the behavior therapy and star chart systems are too complicated and don't work for your family?

You won't find any solutions to these dilemmas in the medical textbooks. Most often, they are found in the accumulated wisdom of parents who have acquired that knowledge, often through the same trial-and-error process that I have had to go through. So this book is not only written by a physician but, more important, it is also infused with the wisdom of the many parents whose experiences have shaped the advice and information in this book—parents who, like you, have spent lots of time in the trenches trying to make it work in the best way possible for themselves, their child, and their unique life circumstances.

Remember, You're Trying to Manage a Chronic Illness

To fill in the long answer to the question, "Why haven't things gotten a lot better for our child with ADHD and our family?", you have to keep in mind that you're dealing with a chronic illness and all its challenges. Many parents forget, because ADHD is classified as a psychiatric disorder rather than as a medical illness, that it's just as difficult to handle as, say, asthma or diabetes. Even with a relatively treatable condition such as asthma, in addition to carefully monitoring your child's medications, you must ensure that baby sitters, teachers, and other relatives know what to do if your child has an attack and you are not there. Now think about the kinds of steps you must take to prevent your child's exposure to potential triggers that can set off an attack, such as house dust, pollens, or pets. To make matters more complex, think about having to leave work and cancel other plans to pick up your child at school and take him or her to the emergency room for assistance during an acute attack.

With either asthma or diabetes, how about the challenges of sending your child off to camp or even only to stay overnight with friends? What other special arrangements will you have to make to make sure it works out OK? And how many times, despite your best efforts, will these steps still not be enough to prevent problems? What special dietary guidelines will your child have to follow? What do you do if he doesn't like these restrictions or "just wants to be like other kids"? What do you do if your child refuses medication?

As if these problems weren't enough, consider the additional burdens you experience when you must face all the assorted red tape machines in our current world, such as the school that says your kid doesn't need special resources, or the insurance company that says your child's ADHD is not covered or that your child cannot see the specialist recommended by your child's primary doctor.

You'd feel a lot of sympathy and compassion for a family dealing with a child's asthma or diabetes. So why not feel a little compassion for yourself and your family's plight? The first step toward understanding why things aren't as good as you believe they should be is to remind yourself that you're up against a ream of tough challenges.

The Double Whammy of ADHD:
A Chronic Childhood Condition with Extra Challenges—
and How This Book Can Help

Like asthma and diabetes, ADHD is a long-term problem requiring a long-term, big-picture strategy if you are to succeed in optimizing your child's treatment program—and life! But it raises some additional problems that chronic medical illnesses often do not. Below I list some of the big-picture issues that we as parents must grapple with. Despite their obvious importance, these are the things I was not taught in medical school or during specialty training and that you need to be aware of, so you can anticipate the problems they may cause. Turn to the chapters mentioned for help in these particular areas.

• *ADHD medicines, while effective, are far from perfect.* The best established, most tested, and most effective medications are the "stimulant" medications involving agents such as various forms of methylphenidate (Ritalin, Concerta, Metadate, Metadate CD, Ritalin LA, Focalin) or amphetamine compounds (Adderall, Adderall XR). Quite clearly, these agents have side effects that can affect the child's appetite, sleep habits, and mood.

Other problems with the current medication treatments are that because they are controlled substances (with abuse potential), they usually require the doctor to write (and the parent to get) a new prescription each month. While new medications have been devel-

> ### What the Textbooks Don't Say
>
> - ADHD medicines aren't perfect
> - Stigma related to ADHD and medicine
> - Difficulties doing behavior therapies
> - Communications with the doctor
> - Insurance companies don't want to pay
> - The school system doesn't want to help
> - Parents disagree about treatment and discipline
> - Your boss doesn't understand why you need to take so much time off
> - Knowing why your child behaves this way doesn't make him more likeable to others
> - Lack of resources in the community
> - Contradictory information and advice
> - Wondering if you're doing the right thing
> - Getting it all done
> - Difficulty accepting the child's problem and planning for the future

oped (such as Strattera) that are not controlled substances, they may not necessarily work for a given child, and stimulant medications are still often needed. *More on these issues in Chapter 5.*

• *Medication treatments (like ADHD itself) are highly stigmatized.* Consider the fact that the current public perception as portrayed in the media is one of shock:

"You're *drugging* your child?!" The rational response, of course, is this one from a wise parent: "Imagine your child has diabetes: Would you refuse to give him insulin? ADHD is a real disease, it is genetic, and the child needs help." So why don't the media and the general public say this to parents whose children have asthma? Or epilepsy? My own feeling is that it is because the general public perception is that ADHD is not a "real problem," but that it is caused by lax parents or overcrowded classrooms. Regardless of the source of stigma, it makes the use of the medications an ongoing source of anxiety and sometimes even guilt for the parents, and something that the child may be concerned about. It also puts parents and others into difficult situations, where we must make special arrangements to ensure the child's privacy and our own, ensure others' comfort or competence in administering the medication in the parent's absence. *You'll find help in advocating for your child and yourself in every chapter that follows.*

• *The behavior therapy is very complicated, hard to apply, and hard to keep up.* This is one of the challenges that many parents and perhaps most teachers have trouble with. It takes a lot of work to mount a full program at home and school, and without a lot of ongoing support and encouragement, it may fall by the wayside or get used only sporadically, both certain ways to limit its effectiveness. What if the teacher doesn't really want to implement the program or feels she doesn't have time? What if you and your spouse disagree on its implementation? What if you can't keep track of all the charts and details? What if you have misgivings because your child seems to be demanding a bribe from you for what should be expected and expectable behavior? *These issues are addressed in Chapters 6 and 7.*

• *You have difficulty communicating with the doctor.* Go figure! Actually, if the truth be known, this is a big and increasing problem, because most doctors nowadays have not been well trained to communicate with the patients, parents, and families. Yes, the doctor is busy, and yes, he is in a hurry, because he's paid to hurry, and in many instances, if he doesn't, it'll come out of his family time that evening. The average pediatric visit is now about thirteen minutes across the country, and managed care forces are trying to get it down below ten minutes. So it's a complicated problem, and most certainly, only a tiny part of it is *your* difficulty communicating with the doctor. But there are in fact things you can do to enhance the two-way communication with the doctor and maximize the chances of your being understood and having a productive two-way exchange. *More on that in Chapter 5.*

• *Insurance companies don't want to pay for ADHD evaluation and treatments.* Unlike other medical illnesses, conditions like ADHD are often not fully or fairly reimbursed. Your company may not reimburse your pediatrician or family doctor to treat your child's ADHD, meaning the doctor has to take time out of other areas that she can bill for, simply carve it out of her hide, or even "make up" or use other billing codes to disguise to the company that she is treating ADHD. Many companies will pay only one-half of the costs for an ADHD or mental health specialists' visit, set lower limits on the total number of visits you can have per year, or require you to use one of their "preferred providers," who may or may not be qualified to evaluate and treat the condition. And one of the other dirty little secrets that often doesn't get enough discussion is that even if the company says it will cover a certain proportion of the costs, you end up being asked to pay much more because the doctor's fee was above the company's allowable limit. If the doctor is reimbursed at about $24 per hour but bills at the "going rate" of $50 for the same time period, guess who will pay the difference? *What you can do about such problems is discussed in Chapter 5.*

• *The school system has a much different agenda than helping children with ADHD.* Basically schools are set up to provide a "one size fits all, cheap as humanly possible" education. This is not because schoolteachers, principals, or administrators don't care (most do), but simply because schools' capabilities and their ultimate mission are ruled by their political realities, budgets, and language of statutes and authorizing legislation. So all personnel across the system are paid, certified, rated, and promoted to the extent to which their charges do well on standardized academic tests. Anything that takes time or resources away from that mission threatens their livelihood. As a result, you will face many natural obstacles whenever you try to get special resources for a child with ADHD, even if providing them seems to require the staff to go only slightly out of their way. Parents who understand this problem and know how to help school personnel deal with this problem so that both of the parties get their respective ends met have a much better chance of getting their child the best school resources available. *You'll learn more about these strategies in Chapter 6.*

• *Parents disagree about the child's treatment, education, and discipline.* Disagreement between parents is hardly restricted to ADHD. But because the management problems are so much greater for parents of a child with ADHD, there are a lot more areas of potential difficulty, stress, perceived unfairness, and supposed blame. To make matters worse, family dynamics are stressed and strained by the child's ADHD. A disciplinary practice that is perfectly reasonable for most children may backfire for a child with ADHD. If one parent appreciates this while the other doesn't, opportunities for friction abound. While not unique to ADHD, the child may also take advantages of parents' differences of opinion or discipline and play one against the other. School-age children may do this inadvertently, but when parents fail to catch on, some older adolescents have been known to refine this skill to con artist levels of mastery. Look out for this one. *Chapter 7 should prove useful.*

• *Your boss doesn't understand why you need to take so much time off.* Here the problems of stigma and public misunderstanding can easily co-conspire to make your work situation very miserable. If your boss knows that your child has a bona fide medical condition, she may be understanding and allow you full use of family or personal leave. But if you have determined that it is best to *not talk* about your child's condition, or if you have discussed it but your boss has negative attitudes about ADHD or mental health issues, this can be tricky and very difficult. While federal laws and most workplace regulations offer some protections for you, no one wants to compromise the work situation just to exercise his or her rights. How do you make your work "work" while still getting your child the help he or she needs? *Chapter 8 offers a number of approaches used by other parents.*

• *Knowing why your child behaves this way doesn't make the scout leader want him in the troop any more than before.* Yes, adults' and others' awareness of the challenges of the child's ADHD sometimes helps a bit, but this doesn't get him or her any more friends or make him or her more likable. What makes this worse in ADHD, compared, say, to asthma or diabetes, is that ADHD seems so inextricably linked to the child's behavior and personality. All of the ADHD behaviors affect what your child does with (or to) others. So how do you negotiate these difficult situations, and when should you cut your losses and move on to find an alternative social setting or set of experiences for your child? *As you'll see in Chapter 8, these are not always easy decisions.*

• *There's a lack of resources in your community—or you can't afford to pay for what is available.* Yes, it is tough to "get blood out of a turnip," but in most cases, what we need is turnip juice. Unfortunately, no community really has sufficient resources, and even when resources are available, they often prove too costly for most of us. The good news is that even if your community has few resources or is far removed from the widely touted experts, there's so much you can do to make a difference for your child. The fancy degree or the prominent name is no guarantee of a competent resource. In most cases, what will make the difference is the expertise you obtain and how you apply it, not getting an evaluation by Dr. So-and-So at Such-and-Such medical center. *If the need to get all this expertise sounds a bit daunting, don't worry—lots of parents have gone before you, as you'll see in Chapters 5 and 6.*

• *You're getting contradictory information and advice from experts and others.* This is a terrible problem for parents, since it is hard to know who is really an expert and who is not. Anyone can claim expertise, publish a book, or host a website. With so much information, especially contradictory information, available, how do you identify the true facts? And how do you know what's right for *your child* as time goes on? Reading this book will teach you when to trust your expert instincts over those of other "experts," and when you should rely on other experts, not just expert professionals but other expert parents as well. *See Chapter 4 to learn how to judge the quality of information that comes to you via various media.*

• *You're frustrated by your own knee-jerk reactions, wondering if you're doing enough or the right thing.* I've often thought that if I meet a parent who doesn't experience feelings of parental guilt on a regular basis, it is my duty as a physician to check for signs of life. We all make mistakes, but there is no mistake you can make with your ADHD child that is irreversible. *Again, a major thrust of this book is to assist you in expanding your expertise in the area, so you'll find many areas of Part II, especially Chapter 7, quite useful.*

• *There's just too much to do to make it all work—I can't get it all done!* This is an understandable reaction that we all have when we face an unknown task. If someone told me all of the specific muscle movements or steps it takes to ride a bike, or even to play a simple video game, and if I had to do it all at once, like you, I would say, "Too complicated, can't be done." Fortunately, it *is* only one step at a time. And if you believe, like I do, that we are in this for the long run, you are going to have lots of chances to practice. Many parents who have been in your shoes and have mastered these steps, largely on their own, want to help other parents like you become more effective more quickly than they were able to. *Throughout this book, you can reap the benefits of their head start and accumulated experiences.*

• *You have difficulty accepting the child's problem and planning for the future.* This is an important struggle for every parent of a child with ADHD. But much more help and support than you probably realize is available and out there. *See Chapters 2, 3, 4, and 9.*

There's no doubt that the preceding list of challenges is an awful lot to handle. The health professions have come a long way in treating kids with ADHD, but the realities of everyday life are pretty much yours to manage. The key is to learn to *make* things work—to work around a strapped school district, to make an overtaxed teacher an ally, to be assertive with doctors, to find that one person at your insurance company who understands that you are a paying customer, to enlist the support that's offered by informal parent groups and national organizations alike, to know where to get the facts on everything from the latest scientific research to your child's legal rights, to special education and disability services. That's what this book is for—to describe how you can make the system work for your child and your family as well as it possibly can. Becoming an expert in making the system work can make all the difference in whether your child and your family not only survive the ordeal but also *thrive* despite the difficulties.

So how prepared are you to do that? The following quiz should help you evaluate whether you as a parent are as effective, expert, and empowered as you can possibly be in getting the best care for your child. No doubt, it will show that in some areas you're already an expert, but if you are feeling frustrated by the problems you've been experiencing with your child's care, it will help you pinpoint possible sources of the trouble and identify the areas in which you might want to focus your energies. If you're just starting out on your journey with ADHD in the family, it will help you head off problem areas from the start.

QUIZ

Are You Making the System Work for You?

1. Do you know how many years of experience your current doctor has with ADHD and how many children with ADHD he or she has treated?

2. Are your household rules fair to all your children?

3. When you have a problem with your child's teacher, do you call the principal first?

4. If a relative questioned whether your child really has ADHD, would you be able

to explain why the diagnosis seems to fit your child—and why other diagnoses do not?

5. When your doctor is rude or curt, do you respond the same way you would respond to a salesperson, your accountant, or your personal trainer?

6. Does your doctor talk about your child in his presence, as if he's not there?

7. If another professional asks for your child's medical records, can you easily pull them from your file in your home office?

8. Do you know whether your child would benefit from untimed testing or homework assignments reduced in length?

9. Do you and your spouse call each other "pushover" or "tyrant," claiming that one of you lets the child with ADHD "get away with murder," while the other is "way too hard" on him or her?

10. Have you asked your child's teacher what you can do at home to follow up on the teacher's efforts to help your child at school?

11. When your insurance company denies a claim or reimburses you insufficiently, do you know how to challenge the decision? Do you get your employer involved in the appeal?

12. Have you discarded star charts because they just didn't work as they were described?

13. Has your doctor ever pointed out a creative way for you to get the best possible care for your child, when it looks as if the limitations of your insurance coverage might stand in the way?

14. Has your child's teacher asked you what you think your child needs most?

15. If there's no ADHD support group in your area, do you just do without support?

16. Do you know whom you are entitled to invite to an individualized education plan (IEP) meeting?

17. If your doctor seems impatient when you want to ask questions at the end of your appointment, do you say that you can see she doesn't have much time right now and ask when you can schedule another visit or phone call just to ask questions?

18. Have you stopped reading your children without ADHD bedtime stories, discontinued the Friday night family Monopoly game, or let your other kids do their homework unsupervised because you're spending so much time with your child with ADHD?

19. Have you ever asked your child's teacher to intervene to stop peer teasing?

20. Can friends come to your home to play with your other children without interference from your child with ADHD?

21. Have you put off your own doctor's appointments because you're so busy taking your child to the doctor?

22. Do you know that you have the right to take a family leave from your job?

23. Do you know other parents of kids with ADHD?

24. If anyone asked you how kids get ADHD, would your instinctive response be to blame yourself?

25. Is there a reporting system by which you and the teacher can keep track of how things are going daily, weekly, and monthly?

26. Can you openly discuss your child's diagnosis with him or her?

27. Do you speak frankly about your child's disorder at home but refer to it as his or her "little problem" everywhere else?

28. Can you approach another parent to discuss it when your child isn't invited to a party?

29. Has the teacher asked for the names of your child's doctor, therapist, and others providing ADHD-related care?

30. Do you keep enrolling your child in different activities, keeping your fingers crossed that eventually he'll find one where he just fits in?

What It Means

If your answers followed the pattern *yes, yes, no* throughout the quiz, you're already an expert parent and may not need this book. The fact that you're reading it anyway only confirms your willingness and ability to take charge of your child's care and get him or her the best treatment out there. Congratulations. (In fact, you can probably add to the tips you'll find in the following pages. I hope you're passing them on to other parents.)

More likely, your answers followed the pattern *no, no, yes*. The more they conformed to this pattern, the more you need this book. Those answers indicate that you may not have the confidence or the knowledge to go after what your child and you need, and that the helping professionals you're working with may not be helping you as much as they could or should. These answers should confirm that you need help, and they should help you figure out where your current strengths and weaknesses lie in serving as manager of your child's care.

Did you answer the questions this way? (Turn to the next page.)

1. No	11. No	21. Yes
2. No	12. Yes	22. No
3. Yes	13. No	23. No
4. No	14. No	24. Yes
5. No	15. Yes	25. No
6. Yes	16. No	26. No
7. No	17. No	27. Yes
8. No	18. Yes	28. No
9. Yes	19. No	29. No
10. No	20. No	30. Yes

Most of the questions—1, 3–5, 7, 8, 10–12, 15–20, 22–24, 26–28, and 30—ask about your actions, because what *you* do is the most powerful determinant of the kind of care your child ends up getting. That's the underlying point of this book. If you answered these questions as listed above, you'll want to polish your ability to deal with the professionals treating your child; rethink your attitudes toward yourself, your ADHD child, and your family; replace blame with responsibility; assert your rights as a consumer of mental healthcare services and parent; and make a permanent commitment to becoming as knowledgeable and savvy as you can—starting with reading this book.

But this quiz can tell you more:

- If you answered questions 6, 12, and 13 as shown above, your helpers in the healthcare system aren't serving you too well; if you answered questions 1, 5, 7, 11, and 17 as shown above, you're not getting all you could from them. In either case, Chapter 5 can help.
- If you answered questions 14, 25, and 29 as shown above, your child's school or teachers may not be up to par; if you answered questions 3, 8, 10, 16, and 19 as shown, you may need to learn how to deal with these providers. I tell you how to solve these problems in Chapter 6.
- For matching answers to questions 9, 18, and 20, or 2, 15, 21, 23, and 26, take advantage of the tips on creating a nurturing home life for the whole family in Chapter 7.
- Likewise, for questions 4, 22, 24, 28, and 30, you'll find a wealth of empowering ideas in Chapter 8.

What You Stand to Gain

If you already feel exhausted and beleaguered, or anxious about the challenges that lie ahead, you may be worried that I'm simply giving you another huge task to complete. Let me remind you that this book is here to do most of the work for you, in the form of tips and support from parents who've already traveled this road. The point is not to take more of your time but to save you time. Also, you can always pick and choose from the following chapters; don't bother with anything that feels like more trouble than it's worth to you. And if you have any doubts about the return you'll get for making any extra effort, listen to what these parents have to say:

> "At first the school didn't want to do anything that was going to cost them money, like tutoring or special support. End of story, so I thought. But the doctor then told me about my son's educational rights under federal legislation. I began to push back. The doctor wrote a letter to the school about my son's educational needs. Things really began to move after I got a lawyer friend to write the school a letter on legal stationery. I'd like to say everything's hunky dory now. It's not. It's better, but I still have to push on the system. But I have a good feel for which buttons to push."

> "My situation may be somewhat different than most. I have been a school board member since my son was six. I was able to get our superintendent to get the special education dept. to identify children with ADHD under 'other health impaired [OHI].' Five years ago there was not one child in our school district of 11,000 with OHI eligibility. As a result of my doing a survey of fifty parents, bringing the info from the survey to our administrators and just plain lobbying them hard, they started identifying our kids. Now there are eighty-five kids with OHI eligibility. Things have improved for many children."

> "Doctors would drop out of my insurance plan. I would change doctors, and finally I was so frustrated, I called one of my old doctors that I really liked. I told him, 'I can't find anybody on the plan.' He said he would negotiate with the insurance company as if he were in their plan. My husband called the insurance company and told them, 'We are having a hard time getting a doctor'—they would not call back; if they did call back and then found out which insurance I had, they made up an excuse that they were not taking any new patients or that they were not with the insurance company anymore. Finally the insurance company agreed to use the doctor I wanted. The insurance company themselves called doctors that were within certain miles of where I lived. They said we were right. They could not get us a doctor either. So now they are paying my doctor $200 for thirty minutes!"

Two

PRINCIPLES OF ACTION FOR THE EXPERT PARENT

"Put your child first and trust your instincts. Don't let anyone make you doubt yourself."

"Educate yourself so that you don't hate yourself or your child by believing people around you who tell you that your child is a juvenile delinquent."

"If you don't agree with your doctor's line of treatment or opinions on this topic, find another doctor."

"Provide a lot of love, patience and understanding."

The idea that finding solutions to your ADHD-related problems initially lies within you can be a bit overwhelming, to be sure. But this realization can actually be quite liberating: Now you can prepare to act, rather than continue to wait for others to act. The battle may be far from over, but you know where your strengths and weaknesses lie, so you're ready to strategize.

It may seem a bit strange to use the term *adversary* here, since your ultimate goal is to get teachers, doctors, relatives, and others to work on behalf of your child. But the current reality is that many of these otherwise well-intentioned persons are putting obstacles in the way of your child's optimal care, and you have to get over or around them to move the battle line forward. This may mean pushing a bit harder than seems natural or comfortable. If so, remember that your goal is not to *defeat* these others who must play a role in your child's healthcare. Rather, it's to *capture* them long enough to turn them into allies. This is not your grandmother's healthcare system, nor your grandfather's one-room schoolhouse. It may not even resemble the kinds of relationships with medical and school personnel that you grew up with. So, in this new landscape, effective battle strategies draw on new principles. The principles discussed in this chapter represent parents' accumulated wisdom. These are the fallback tenets that they urge you to keep in mind when the going gets rough and your specific tactics don't seem to be working. They should form the foundation of the strategies you devise and serve collectively as your care management mantra.

1. You're in Charge

This principle is essential, because it's the foundation for all the principles that follow. Yet it might not be easy to adopt, because all of us have grown up in the culture of "doctor knows best." The doctor is the expert, the teacher is a certified professional, the therapist has had years of training. But it is your child, not theirs. Your child has legal rights in the educational and healthcare system, and it is your role to exercise these rights on behalf of your child. Sometimes the system may fail your child, not because other people don't care, but simply because they have different tasks and responsibilities. The teacher is in charge of the classroom, but you are in charge of your child. The doctor is responsible for providing sound medical advice, but in most (but not all) instances you are in charge of deciding whether to accept that advice or to seek out a second opinion, if the first one doesn't make sense to you. Similarly, get used to the fact that eventually you are likely to know more about ADHD than your child's teacher, and you will definitely know more about how your child learns best and what kinds of school accommodations will work best for your child.

> **Principles of Action for the Expert Parent**
>
> 1. You're in charge.
> 2. Don't be intimidated.
> 3. You are not responsible for your child's illness.
> 4. Everyone works for you.
> 5. You know your child best.
> 6. Informed is armed.
> 7. There are no dead ends.
> 8. No expectation or goal is written in stone.
> 9. You're not infallible.
> 10. You need and deserve support.
> 11. There's life beyond your child's ADHD.
> 12. Take care of yourself.
> 13. Learn to let go.

Being in charge does not mean doing it all, of course, any more than being the boss means doing everyone's job. You should not need to devise accommodations for your child in the classroom, for example; you should learn about the various possible accommodations supported by federal law that a classroom teacher might make to facilitate the learning of a child with ADHD. (Chapter 6, plus Appendix A of this book, is a good place to start, but for additional details of what is available in your district, you'll want to contact your school district's Section 504 coordinator at the district's headquarters. Ask for the Assistant Superintendent or Director of Special Education Services, and request their available written materials for parents detailing the district's Section 504 options.) Where you take charge is in making sure your child gets the services that you feel, knowing your child as thoroughly as you do, are appropriate. Let's say the teacher does not want to make any seating rearrangements to move your child to the front of the class, while you, in fact, know that your child is likely to benefit from that. If you don't know your child's legal rights, or you're intimidated by the teacher, you might stay silent, feeling you've hit a dead end. Or your frustration might make you feel so angry that you make aggressive demands that only alienate the teacher. Becoming knowledgeable and learning how to communicate effectively will allow you to take this approach with the teacher, if push comes to shove: "I know how terribly disruptive this must be for your class and other students, but we really need to find a way to work this out or to find some other equally helpful arrangements." Notice that this parent showed understanding of the teacher's plight, used the *we* word, offered to participate in coming up with a solution, and adopted a pleasant tone of voice and an understanding nod. Being in charge means being firm and direct without being hostile, as well as taking responsibility rather than laying blame. "Things are better because I'm a dedicated parent who is proactive," said one mother. "I must keep in close contact with my child's teachers and spend a lot of time coordinating her daily work so that she can be successful." It's your right as a parent to be in charge; this book will give you the skills to do it right.

Too often, as parents of kids with ADHD, you may end up feeling like you are not in charge at all—that you're at the mercy of the child's unpredictable, impulsive behavior, trapped in the chaos of a child's hyperactivity, stuck trying to motivate the kid to stay on task, all of which can rob parents of confidence: "What am I doing wrong?" you ask. Or maybe you feel worn down by how school staff treat your child or you. Yes, it is very hard to stay in charge and calm and pleasant when you're frustrated and angry. In later chapters, particularly Chapters 5, 6, and 7, we'll role-play various approaches to this problem and give you other ideas and tips for how to do this.

"Our daughter cannot be with us all day," noted one parent. "We rely on many others to medicate her, ensure that she is mentally healthy, and guide her throughout her day at school." Her solution? Establish a board of directors: pediatrician, psychologist, teachers, school counselor, tutor.

2. Don't Be Intimidated

Like it or not, most professionals have learned to act with certainty in the face of uncertainty. The teacher has to have a lesson plan for your child, whether it fits or not. The doctor has to form an opinion and make recommendations on the basis of cursory information. While that might work well with strep throat, it doesn't work nearly as well with complex issues of development, where your instincts may tell you something else. So don't be intimidated by the professional's seeming certainty. You're a professional too—a professional parent! You are your child's best and most effective advocate, and that ultimate responsibility can be handled by no one else nearly as effectively as you.

Imagine for the moment that you have been told by your child's doctor that you shouldn't worry about some problem your child is having, perhaps with the doctor's prescribed treatment, such as the effects of medication on sleep or appetite. Well, they *are* your worries, not the doctor's, and just having some "expert" say one thing or the other does not always make it so. What do you do? Simply, you need to be comfortable asserting yourself further and not back off when that is against your better judgment. For your own peace of mind, and for the benefit of your child, it is usually better to hang in there, persist with voicing your question or concern, until there has been sufficient discussion that you feel comfortable with the final solution arrived at by you and the doctor.

Many of the parents I've gotten to know over the years are great models for being assertive when dealing with ADHD experts and other professionals. "Don't listen to only one person or public school personnel," advises one mother. Throughout this book, parents tell you how they resisted feeling intimidated by professionals, and I'll show you some methods for honing your assertiveness. Persistence pays.

3. You Are Not Responsible for Your Child's Illness

Not only do we often blame ourselves for our child's problems, but others may also spring this trap as well. One mother's experience may sound all too familiar: "In kindergarten, my son's experienced teacher told me he was a behavior problem and did not have ADHD: 'You are doing something wrong at home.' I took him for a diagnosis the following summer and changed schools. Wow! What a difference." Because educational and medical professionals often form opinions in the face of little information (don't blame them; that's their job), they sometimes reach wrong conclusions. This happens especially often in complex areas and where there is some degree of uncertainty, such as ADHD. And one common but very disconcerting conclusion is that somehow you are to blame for your child's problems. You're not strict enough. You and your spouse need to work together better and agree on your parenting approaches. Your husband or wife shouldn't travel so much or should work shorter hours. You should quit your job. You should spend more quality time with your child. You shouldn't be so hard on your child. And so on. Here's how to react, in the simple words of one experienced parent: "Don't blame yourself or let anyone make you feel responsible for your child's illness."

Also watch out for blame cloaked as advice.

"The school nurse told us that our child just needed some good spankings. In-laws also suggested minor beatings. We were told that he behaved this way because he was eating sugar—or because of the food dyes in his food. (All blamed me, Mom, for not punishing him or for not being smart enough to feed him well, in spite of the fact that I had a home economics degree and had studied child development and nutrition.) Most people seemed to delight in telling us how awful he was and what we should do about it. Everyone seemed to be an 'expert'—but none of them made any positive suggestions that could help."

Of course, as parents, we are responsible for our child's care, but research has shown that parents do not cause ADHD. So it isn't just a "discipline problem" (i.e., it's your fault), even though these kids are a big discipline problem (yes, it's your challenge!). It's very easy for someone who doesn't live with your child twenty-four hours a day, seven days a week, to reach wrong conclusions. In such instances, for the less than optimally informed professional, the easiest conclusion to reach is one that doesn't involve any activity or new effort on his part. *You* should change, not your child. That's where you come in, and where a battle line *sometimes* will need to be drawn. But remember, winning a battle doesn't always require a frontal assault. In fact, that will be the least effective strategy in many instances. More about handling such problems later.

4. Everyone Works for You

Yes, you pay for the doctor's salary. Your taxes or your tuition pay the teacher's salary. It's their job to work on your child's behalf, and their professional codes require that of them. This doesn't mean that you want to act entitled or demanding, though there are times when you must push. Instead, it means that you should feel and ex-ude a quiet confidence that, of course, they will take whatever necessary steps they must to ensure your child's best health outcomes. When you feel it, this quiet confidence means that you will be slow to anger if they are less than well informed, tolerant but insistent, just as you would with a new employee. As a good employer and manager, you won't want to lose your temper quickly. You will appreciate that your new employees need time to learn about you and your child, what the job entails, what your expectations are, and so forth.

Sometimes we get this all turned around, as do those with whom we must interact concerning our children. For example, one of the more humorous statements I sometimes hear when providing guidance to teachers or doctors on best procedures to apply is, "But I'm a *professional*!" Essentially this means, "I know what I am doing, I answer to no one, so don't try to tell me what to do." Whether "I am a professional" is stated explicitly or not, remember that you (or your taxpayer dollars, no matter) in essence employ this person, and you need to get his or her assistance in getting the best for your child. Don't settle for less. Parents of a kid with ADHD can end up feeling like they're in a real one-down position because their child's symptoms require a lot of intervention and can cause disruption wherever the child interacts with others. It might not be so hard for you to feel like "the boss" when your only "hired help" is a pediatrician, but add to your staff a special education teacher, a therapist, maybe a child psychiatrist, and others, and it's like starting out supervising a staff of twelve on your very first job.

Throughout this book, with lots of input from the parents who've been there before, I show you how to get comfortable in this new role. For example, imagine that a teacher or doctor hears your request for a specific type of assistance for your child but feels it is not necessary and responds, "Mrs. Smith, you are just going to have to trust me as a professional." With practice, and through this book, you will learn how to reply; for example, "I do appreciate all of your training, but as Johnnie's parent, I have a lot of experience, and I am pretty expert with his needs. So we need to find a way to work together, blending our knowledge, and put together a plan that works for him."

5. You Know Your Child Best

I can't tell you how often I've heard this story: Parents repeatedly see their son lose focus and fail to remember instructions they have given; they're hoarse from the frequent reminders they've had to issue for their child to complete assigned tasks. Yet the child appears to pay attention just fine in the doctor's office, and the well-intentioned doctor says, "He's just fine" or "It's just a phase," only to find out later that the phase never ended or it only led to worse difficulties. (As you may already know, this phenomenon is a direct result of the nature of ADHD: In a new and possibly intriguing setting, your child may be perfectly able to sit still and pay attention because he's currently engrossed.) Although teachers, doctors, coaches, and others may have valuable insight about your child, by and large, you know your child better than any of them. The teacher has only passing knowledge of up to thirty children, and then only in a very specific kind of setting. Divide the teacher's six-hour day with the class by thirty kids, and the teacher is spending the equivalent of twelve minutes a day with your child. On average across the country, your doctor may see your child for only two fifteen-minute sessions a year. None of them will be as aware as you are likely to be of your child's moods, self-esteem, likes and dislikes, fears, and hopes. Your gut instincts are critical and should be trusted.

The opinions of these other "players" counts as well, of course, because doctors, teachers, coaches, and others have the benefit of seeing many children at once in group settings and are often able to compare what is "normal" or not among the children. But parents will be more aware of subtle clues that may not show up in the doctor's office. So listen to your gut—but also listen to others, and seek their opinions and input. If there is uncertainty about how to address the problem, get more information, using some of the approaches I talk about in Chapter 4. If multiple sources are telling you the same thing, even when it goes against your gut, remember to apply the modesty principle to your own opinions as well.

6. Informed Is Armed

So much more information is available nowadays to parents than ever before. But this is a double-edged sword. With so much often conflicting information, how do you know what's right? "Don't believe Peter Breggin [who claims that ADHD is not a genuine diagnosis] and all the Scientologists' anti-Ritalin propaganda," advises one parent. "Don't buy into the 'indigo child' [a child who displays new or unusual attributes that require special treatment and upbringing to achieve harmony in their lives] crap either. Do extensive research before buying any product or starting any diet that claims to 'cure' ADHD."

So you will need to do some homework. Learn all you can about ADHD, your local community resources, and the latest research. Fortunately, you will not be alone in this, and there are many reputable websites, government agencies (your tax dollars!), healthcare professional groups, and local and national parent organizations that spend a lot of dollars to review the latest information and make it available at no cost. Here are some of the sources parents have learned to rely on:

- "The biggest gift of all is the National CHADD Organization. They educated me about the condition through collecting the best national researchers and authorities on ADHD each year at the conference. I have been able to hear the results of the latest research over the last sixteen years."
- "Read everything you can get your hands on that is written by credible researchers and authorities on ADHD and other mental health issues."
- "I spent some time on a message board at *Ivillage.com*, parent soup—that was for parents who have children with attention deficit disorder (ADD)/ADHD."
- "Our state family resource center for disabled kids has been a godsend, as has the state Office of Exceptional Learners." Do you know about these resources in your state? If not, see Chapter 4.
- "For services not offered in the private school I used the state Child Find program for speech therapy for both of my children." There are counterparts for this program in every state. Although resources and eligibility will vary from state to state, these may be helpful to you. See Chapter 4.
- "I received very helpful advice from a local child advocacy group." Which are available in your area? See Chapter 4 for how to find this out.
- "The biggest difference to us has been the age of technology. When my child was little, I couldn't find enough information on the subject. Now, I can access any medical college's library, any medical journal, and any written information online. What a real help in getting the information I need!"
- "What's made a difference to me has been reading various resources, including and especially *Attention!* magazine."

You'll find a lot more suggestions for finding helpful resources in Chapters 3 and 4.

7. There Are No Dead Ends

We all get stuck sometimes and think there is no way out. This certainly happens to parents trying to get care for their children with ADHD. What if the teacher or school says "No way!" to what you think is a reasonable request? What if the doctor is not available? What if the treatment doesn't seem to be working? What if you have "tried everything"? Solutions to such problems are never easy or ideal, but almost always there is something you can do to take charge and get yourself or your child out of the corner. In my experience, the illusion that you've reached a dead end is almost always created by a loss of the big picture. You can no longer see or fully appreciate the corner you're in or the way out. In such situations, biding your time, watching for the storm to break, and moving ahead when conditions are favorable may be a good strategy. Most often, though, consulting with others is better. Other parents are frequently the single best sources of information and guidance in these situations.

The bottom line is, you can get where you need to be from where you are. Nothing is irretrievable or inevitable (except death and taxes?), and solutions not apparent now will eventually reveal themselves. Continued problem solving and perseverance are key. Your child's ADHD is not a problem you can just "fix," and you have to remember that you're in this for the long haul. This is not a sprint. It's a cross-country trek, and you'll have many opportunities along the way to make course corrections or even to double back if needed. You will make parenting mistakes. The treatments will rarely be perfect. Your child's teacher may not be ideal. (In fact it's extremely common to hear a parent say something like "Last year his teacher had unrealistic expectations and he spent the whole year feeling like a failure," followed by something like: "Having a great teacher this year in school has made a tremendous difference. This year his teacher goes above and beyond to help him succeed and even celebrates with him when he accomplishes a task." As for kids without ADHD, sometimes your child will have a great teacher, some years a not-so-great one. It's rare for a child to have terrible teachers year after year.) But if you view the landscape from above, many of these problems are temporary or only small "blips" on the radar screen. This means you should pick your battles carefully, whether with your child, the school system, or even family members. The "Custer's last stand" approach to working with the system and various obstacles along the way can backfire, both personally, as you exhaust yourself trying to solve a problem, and by alienating those whose efforts you need on behalf of your child.

Some of the *apparent* dead ends that you are likely to encounter repeatedly are (1) the lack of knowledge or stigmatizing attitudes among those persons (e.g., doctors, teachers) who *should* know about ADHD and *should* be able to help but don't; (2) the simple lack of resources in many school systems; and (3) the fact that some insurance companies either won't pay for ADHD or drag their feet every step of the way. There are way too many of these obstacles strewn along your course, so you have to decide carefully which supposed dead end you should tackle, and tackle first. More on that in Chapter 3, on planning.

Because it is a marathon, you need to conserve resources and use them wisely. That means filling up the tank well before you have run out of fuel. One thing I have learned in running almost twenty marathons is that it is essential to drink water or a sport drink at every water-hole opportunity, usually every three miles in most marathons. If I wait until I *notice* that I'm thirsty, it's too late. By the time I notice my thirst, I cannot drink enough to restore what I have lost and still run a good race. So you may feel OK right now, but if you don't take care of yourself and make sure you prevent yourself from getting depleted, you won't be there when your child still needs you. More on taking care of yourself in Chapter 7.

Remember also, because it is a marathon, that it is not supposed to be easy. Marathons are challenging and can take a lot out of you. But because you're going to pace yourself along the way, making sure you don't get to the point of exhaustion, you can endure some pain. Your child is worth it, and you will be glad, not just when you have crossed the finish line but even along the way.

"The best advice I've ever gotten came from a book, *ADHD and Teens*, by Colleen Alexander-Roberts," said one parent. "In it she says that while it is easy to feel like a bad parent, remember that if you are doing *anything* that is targeted at helping your child with his or her ADHD, then you are *not* a bad parent. Remembering that when things seem to be going badly really helps!"

8. No Expectation or Goal Is Written in Stone

Sometimes we take ourselves and our plans a bit too seriously, and we forget that flexibility is critical. You always have the right to change your mind, and you may have to do so when circumstances change. Yes, the consistency that's so often stressed in parenting a child with ADHD is important, but it should not be a substitute for logic and flexibility.

Because our son with ADHD was a bright kid, my wife, Suzy, and I were adhering to the straightforward notion that it was a good thing for him to apply himself and develop his talents. So in fifth grade, he had the option to be in an advanced, "gifted and talented" class. We enrolled him and he started, but before long, it was clear he didn't want to continue. Bad idea, we thought. We were reluctant to let him stop, since we thought (fairly simplistically) that that would teach him bad habits (i.e., all you have to do is complain, and your parents will bail you out). Well, Suzy persevered to get me to be more open-minded about the situation, so we met with his "gifted and talented" teacher.

In our meeting, we were shocked to learn that her idea of the best way to teach the kids was to show those smart kids that they weren't so smart after all! She gave them problems that were designed to stump them, so that they would see what it was like to have to struggle. This was like mixing oil and water, as far as my son's already fragile self-esteem was concerned. So throwing consistency to the wind, and thinking more about his immediate self-esteem and the lack of clear-cut value to this exercise in frustration, we pulled him from the class. He was a lot happier, and so were we. And it didn't hurt him one bit. He didn't grow up always trying to get out of things by complaining.

So remember, consistency is a good principle, but it's not the only one. If you make a rule and then realize the rule doesn't make sense, acknowledge it.

Successful outcomes for kids (and families!) come not from consistency as much as from clarity, flexibility, and individualizing what we do for the needs of the given child at a given time in a given situation. Our children are developing and maturing all the time, and our expectations need to reflect what's new. What may work for the child at age six will not work at age seven or eight. What worked for the oldest child may not work for the second child.

9. You're Not Infallible

A corollary to principle 8 is that you're going to make mistakes. I've learned that the best way to correct such mistakes is to start by apologizing, especially when it's your child who was right and you were wrong. ADHD can provoke a lot of anger and frustration. If you find yourself directing it at your child, you're only human. And as long as your response is within reason and aimed at a specific situation, it will serve as part of how the child learns to be responsible and responsive to the needs of others. If, on the other hand, your emotional reaction is disproportionate, inappropriate, or violent, don't be afraid to seek professional advice. You'll be in good company, and I personally have found such help extremely valuable for me at multiple points in my own parenting.

Also remember that none of us is infallible in managing our children's healthcare. You may take some wrong turns here and there. You may try medication and find out it doesn't work that well for your child. You may choose a therapist that ends up not being very good for your child. You may decide that you've been too strict with your child. Get used to it; it's part of the territory. Fortunately, in almost all cases, there's no real harm done. You might feel you've lost time, but, in fact, time is on your side, because you have the opportunity to work out better solutions over the next weeks, months, and even years.

10. You Need and Deserve Support

When I asked parents what has made the biggest difference in their learning to handle problems related to ADHD, virtually all of them named other parents. "CHADD made me realize I was not alone," said one woman. "I found other moms that were going through the same thing. We exchanged phone numbers—and spent a lot of time on the phone together. These moms are located literally all over the world. Some have truly become 'sisters'—we've traveled to share time together." Said another, "Without a doubt, the most helpful thing for me has been connecting with other parents who also have children with ADHD. It is great to be able to hear how they have used different strategies that could be used with my son."

Raising a child, especially one with ADHD, is very hard work, and it is almost impossible to do alone. Other parents who are struggling with the same problems you are can offer ideas for handling sticky issues, support for the emotional upheaval of dealing with a child's chronic illness, and simple camaraderie when you need it. If your child has just been diagnosed, look for a support group (a good place to begin is with CHADD) right away; see Chapter 4 and the information in Appendix B on how to find these and other resources. You may not think you need it right now, but you'll be surprised by the information and services you can benefit from.

Of course, if you have a spouse, and your spouse is supportive of your role, lucky you. In such cases, it is important to talk about the challenges, to trade off with each other when one of you needs a break. Learn each other's strengths and weaknesses and see if you can work to complement each other. In our own family, I have generally been the one who provides structure, limits, and goal setting with the children, while my wife has been especially good at providing one-on-one support, patience, and understanding. This has been especially important for our son with ADHD; her abundant patience has benefited him greatly and has complemented my ability to provide structure and help him set goals. Fortunately, both of us have been able to teach and learn from each other, so that we have not only complemented but also strengthened each other.

Sometimes the significant other adult in your life just doesn't get it. As one woman described it, "My husband said he didn't believe in ADHD. I felt so alone." In a case like that, the important thing is to find someone you can turn to. It may not be someone you are close to, but it should be someone "who gets it." It might be a child care worker, a teacher, a coworker, or a wise secretary. For example, at one point when I was struggling with one of my children, my boss's secretary, a grandmother with lots of experience, reassured me and gave me some confidence that what I was experiencing during my child's teenage rebellion was going to be time-limited. The point is, you might find support where you least expect it, just as I did. Take it where you can get it.

The key is to make sure what you're getting is true support, not a Monday morning quarterback who wants to second-guess and criticize everything you do. Maybe your child's grandparent, an uncle or aunt, or a close friend of yours will be a good candidate—someone in whom you can confide, who won't judge you and simply point out your mistakes. If you feel better and unburdened after talking with this person, he or she could be a good source of support. You need someone who's either really on the team or is waiting for you on the sidelines. If you don't have a truly positive source of support, see Chapter 4.

11. There's Life Beyond Your Child's ADHD

When you're struggling to get things lined up and working better for your child, it probably seems like that is all you have time for. The effort you expend here can be exhausting, and you may feel you have little energy or time left for anything or anyone else. Look out. It has been shown, and is well known, for example, that parents of children with a chronic disorder have more marital problems and are more likely to break up. Why? We don't know for sure, but in part it surely must have something to do with the increased stress and financial burdens. But another part of this is that when we are under stress, a natural response is to retreat emotionally, perhaps to save energy or because we are exhausted. In so doing, other relationships can suffer, and we inadvertently also cut off potential sources of support. Under such conditions, misunderstandings flourish and resentment easily festers for reasons real or imagined.

Not only do marriages suffer under such conditions but siblings of children with chronic illness such as ADHD can also feel the toll. More time may be required for the child with ADHD, and other children may feel things are unfair, or that everyone has to accommodate this child's special needs. Clearly, your relationship with your child with ADHD is not the only relationship that deserves attention. If you look at the big picture, in the long run, all of these other relationships count, so finding a way to invest in them regularly is essential.

Other aspects of life may seem to fade into the background behind ADHD, but do what you can to bring them back into full relief. There are your own interests—the things you did to give your life meaning before ADHD seemed to take over. There are friends, acquaintances, and coworkers who have a lot to offer. You may benefit from giving your time and energies to others besides your child with ADHD, or you may have routes to spirituality that revitalize you. Take a good look at your life and see what aspects you've let go and now miss. You deserve to get them back, even it's just to choose one and carve out time for it.

12. Take Care of Yourself

Reclaiming the important aspects of your life that you've let go in favor of taking care of your child with ADHD is one way to take care of yourself. Get a sitter. Take some time for yourself, and don't feel guilty about it. You need to recharge your batteries to remain in top shape for this continued long trek. So get a life! Remember to enjoy small things on a daily basis. Burnout is a great danger, especially for parents of a child with ADHD. Replenish yourself regularly to avoid burnout. Think of whatever really relaxes you. Get a massage, get a sitter, take a bath, do your nails.

13. Learn to Let Go

Part of the great challenge in avoiding burnout, perhaps even the single greatest challenge throughout this book, is in really accepting your situation and letting go. When I say "letting go," I mean letting go of the fond hope that we can just wave a magic wand and make our child's problems go away. Even if you do everything in this book, your son or daughter is still going to have a hard time . . . still going to be misunderstood by peers or adults . . . still going to be treated unfairly . . . still going to get in trouble at the drop of a hat . . . still going to exasperate you and even frustrate the very efforts intended to help her.

This, as so many parents attest, is one of the most difficult things to face about a child with ADHD:

> "For me it was hardest to first realize that I was dealing with a child with a true disability. Not just a 'difficult' child. Once I accepted this, I was better able to educate myself on all areas of my child's life that would be affected by the disability."

"The hardest thing about accepting my daughter's ADHD was realizing and try-ing to accept that she will always have difficulty in school, making and keeping friends, and watching her struggle through everyday life. As parents we want to shelter our children from any difficulty that they may face."

"For me the hardest thing has been her inappropriate behavior, the lack of con-trol—both her own lack of control and my inability to control her. Then there's the embarrassment in social situations—being judged by others as a parent . . . the feeling of loss at not having a perfect child."

"Letting go" means that deep down, each of us has found a secret, quiet inner place where we have accepted all of these things, where we have accepted ourselves and our child, despite all the many problems that will probably never completely go away. "Letting go" means you still feel you're a good and capable parent, that your child, too, is good and capable.

In effect, what I am talking about is a bit of psychological judo. It's like we have to work with the weight of this problem, allowing it to push us back, and just as we are falling, do a quick sidestep and let it roll over our shoulder. Somehow, we have to be able to reach the point where we can say, "It's OK that she has ADHD. We'll get by. It'll be good enough." Reaching and accepting this position will give us the ability to know when to tackle a problem head on, when to go around it, and when to hold off and wait to fight another day.

This is a tough place to reach, but just as one parent who got there said to me, "It's not that I am *glad* that he has ADHD. It's just that it has refocused our lives, made us more aware of what we have and don't have . . . what we *think* we need and what we *really* need." Or consider what another parent said: "I had to drop out of the rat race. I didn't realize I was in it, but I just couldn't stay on the other treadmill that I was on before. Something had to give, so I did. And although it is not easy, and sometimes I still cry and get mad, I think I have found some more peace with all of this."

I remember one situation with my son, when my frustration was so extreme I thought I would explode. I had decided to become a Scoutmaster as a means of working with and helping my son and, eventually, his two younger brothers. Quality father–son time, right? So after getting under way, finishing Scout Leader training, and beginning with this troop of twenty rambunctious boys, I found out that my most difficult "problem" Scout was my own son, who not only made dealing with him a challenge but also actively undermined the activities I was responsible for helping the other nineteen boys with! There was nothing I could do. I was trapped, down to every last detail and doubly frustrated because it was my son that was putt-ing me in this spot. I was so angry and full of overwhelming feelings. So what did I do? First I shared my feelings with Suzy and had a good long cry. Then I went on a very long walk–run. Two hours' worth. And I let go. I let *something* go, because by the time I returned to the house, I was willing to accept the particular problem my son had thrust on me, and it no longer derailed me—at least, not nearly as much. So I let go of that problem and stopped trying to fix it, because there was no way I could. I gave up trying to control everything that happened to my son. It was good enough just to be his Scoutmaster during those activities; I didn't have to feel (or behave) like a father with a disobedient son in a very public setting. In those situations, I began to respond to him just as I would to my other challenging scouts (as it all turned out, he was not the most challenging!). He, too, was an independent party, and if he didn't like my solutions to his problems, my solutions were not going to work, most definitely not, particularly as he got older.

So remember, the path that you think you need to be on may not be the one you had originally envisioned. But sometimes you need to just hang on and try to enjoy the ride. In fact, this book's goal and its specific approach is to give you what you need to accomplish the most you can accomplish and then move on, so that you can come as close as possible to fulfilling all your desires for your child and family, without draining the very lifeblood out of you and the rest of the family in the process.

From Principles to Planning

The ultimate, most important purpose of all these principles is to give you the critical flexibility and balance—your own personal psychological judo—so that you can, first, stay healthy, care for yourself, and remain in this psychologically balanced judo position; second, move ahead at an appropriate, not too fast pace in implementing a plan for your child; and third, be willing and able to step back and reconnoiter as often as needed, making any useful midcourse corrections to your plan, even including putting it on the shelf, if necessary. Now it's time to formulate a plan.

Three

DEVELOPING A PLAN FOR YOUR CHILD

How to Use Your Knowledge of Yourself and Your Child to Get the Best Care Available

"Initially I blamed myself for not doing more, for not seeing that there was a problem earlier. But it was hard to accept because I had tried to do everything right . . . eating right and taking care of myself after I got pregnant. I looked around and got the best pediatrician I could find. I stopped work for two years, until he was comfortable in day care. I was a maniac in screening his daycare and preschool teachers. This was not supposed to happen. I thought, 'What had I done wrong?' I had to get past all of that stuff before I could really begin to deal with his problems."

"Once I classified my child in my own mind (after being in denial for a few years), I then had to be committed to research, medication therapy, behavioral therapy, educational assistance, planning ahead, etc. So once acceptance set in, I was able to deal with his problems in a different way."

"Financially, it has been hard. We have taken our kids to tutors on and off, but it is worth it. Especially now that my son was accepted into college. I never thought he would be able to go. It has been a long haul, but our efforts seem to be paying off."

The first mother quoted above had obviously gone to great lengths to think through how she was going to raise her son. When her son ended up diagnosed with ADHD, she felt she had failed as a parent. Obviously her parenting did not cause her son's ADHD, but her thinking does illustrate a pitfall I've seen many parents (and others) stumble into. Parents today are especially diligent about setting their children on a path to adult success, but it's as if their plan for raising the child and the realities of what actually happens in the family run on parallel tracks.

Whether it's low academic achievement, social problems, or health challenges, parents end up wondering how trouble has befallen their child when they've worked so hard to give him or her all the advantages. Life just delivers these blows sometimes, of course. But in many cases, the problem is that our plans for our children take on a life of their own. We fail to take into account our child's capabilities and desires, our own strengths and weaknesses, and the family's resources, time pressures, and conflicting priorities. In that case, our plans usually fail because they don't reflect the realities of the child and family, including circumstances, needs, and desires that change over time.

That time element is especially important. Getting what your child needs can take so much effort that you're understandably reluctant to face the fact that those needs have changed. But plans that don't change with the child and family won't serve you well for long.

The best plans keep things moving forward but are realistic, flexible, and feasible considering the resources available to put them into effect. In this chapter, I help you plan in a way that will give you the best possible chance of making the system work for your child. This means first understanding the importance of an overall plan. Many of us would rather skip what sounds like extra work, and we are more inclined to develop a plan once we fully grasp the benefits of doing so. It means establishing short-, intermediate-, and long-term goals, so you can set priorities and use your time wisely. Third, you'll need to identify resources required to reach your objectives, and match your objectives with the necessary resources. Finally, you'll put it all together into a *strategic plan* for the accomplishment of your long-term objectives and an *action plan* for shorter term objectives.

Like the second parent quoted above, if you commit to planning, you'll be able to tackle a formidable set of demands that ADHD presents. And like the third parent quoted, you may find that knowing what your child needs and taking one small step at a time toward it will get you to destinations you never dreamed were possible.

The Impact of Planning:
If You Fail to Plan, You Plan to Fail

Planning won't solve all your problems, but it certainly helps to be prepared for the challenges ahead, just as it helps to store emergency storm supplies if you live in hurricane territory. But planning ahead makes sense for less obvious reasons, too. Psychologically, it's better to take charge of your fate than to passively accept it. Back in the 1960s and 1970s, researchers studied monkeys in pairs, with each pair receiving a small painful stimulus. One monkey, called the "executive monkey," learned that it could push some levers to avoid the pain. If it did so on time, neither monkey in the pair would receive the painful stimulus. The other monkey couldn't do anything. It just had to accept whatever punishment was doled out to the executive monkey. Guess what? This second, "yoked" monkey showed far more signs of stress than the executive monkey, apparently because the executive monkey could *control* its fate, while the yoked monkey could not. In other animal studies, there was a painful stimulus that the animal could not avoid. What happened to such animals? The investigators found these animals developed what they called "learned helplessness," much akin to depression; they withdrew, became more passive, and did not take advantage of other opportunities.

In a sense, effective planning is like taking control, becoming the "executive monkey." From studies of humans, we know that people differ in how they cope with difficult situations. Some of us have a tendency to feel more at the mercy of the difficult situation and give up, while others tend to feel that the same problem is more controllable and make more active efforts to address the problem. It's no surprise which group does better, not just emotionally but also in terms of effectiveness in actually solving the problem. And not planning, not taking control, and just trying to suffer through a difficult situation may actually make us feel worse, more overwhelmed, and less in control. Planning, then, is an essential ingredient for taking charge of your child's care and getting your child and family life onto an even keel. Let's talk about how to do it.

Setting Goals and Objectives

Every well-thought-out plan has one or more goals and objectives, right? What are yours? I would guess they have something to do with getting your child the best care possible. But what does that really mean? This global, overall goal is not very specific. Of course, you want your child to get the best care possible. That's one of the definitions of being a parent! But what does your child need? What are his greatest needs? To set appropriate goals and objectives for our child's care and well-being, we need to know our child's starting points. And goals are like deciding to drive a long cross-country distance on a map, say, from Seattle to Syracuse. We have to know we are in Seattle rather than San Francisco, or none of the maps will make sense. And to really make it to Syracuse, more than just a destination on a map, we need to break this goal into smaller steps: how far we will drive each day and where our stopping points will be, what time we will start off in the morning, and how far we will go before we first stop. Knowing our child's needs is like figuring out where we are on the map.

What Are Your Child's Needs?

Sensible goals must be based on an accurate understanding of your child's needs and strengths. For example, setting unachievable goals, like pushing for a college education for a child/youth who cannot master difficult academic tasks by virtue of the severity of his ADHD or low intelligence, will do everyone a great disservice. Underestimating a child's ability is likely to cause problems as well.

Uncertainties about the right steps to take for *your* child are best dispelled by solid knowledge of your child's needs. Yes, you likely know your child better than anyone else, but others may have special knowledge that you do not—even about your child! Studies have shown many times that parents are unaware of a lot of things about their child. For example, most kids—teenagers—experiment with alcohol and sexual behavior, but parents usually don't know about it. What do you really know about your child? What do you think you don't know for certain but suspect to be the case?

At a basic level, what is your child's overall intelligence? Is he or she gifted? About average? Average? Below average? Which areas might be above average, and which are below average? If your child struggles in reading, does she have offsetting strengths in math? What are his greatest strengths in terms of personal abilities? In the outdoors and nature? Or does your child have good abilities to make friends, or abilities at soccer, swimming, or art? Knowing both your child's strengths and weaknesses is critical, because one time-tested strategy involves capitalizing on those strengths (whatever they are, they may be *the* essential sources of your child's self-esteem), and at the same time building up the weaknesses.

For example, helping the child find and stay involved in an area he can succeed in can be a good long-term strategy. What are those areas of strength? Which areas could be developed and might need special nurturing, for example, through tutoring, extra activities, or lessons, such as additional sports coaching? For our own son, we found that some extra time with a batting coach over several summers was very useful for helping him feel good about his baseball skills. Likewise, basketball camp during the summer helped hone his abilities, so that he didn't get as discouraged during the season. He certainly spent less time on the bench as a result, even though he was not a star. But he was our star, and to himself he was "good enough" that he felt OK.

Things to Know about Your Child: Examples

- What does he like most about himself? Dislike?
- Best academic subject? Worst?
- Intelligence: above average, average, below average?
- What are her greatest areas of natural ability?
- Does he think he is good in sports? School? At? Music?
- Best friend? Why? Least favorite classmate, and why?
- What does she worry most about?
- What is the happiest thing that ever happened to him? The saddest? The scariest?
- What does she want to do or be when she grows up? Why? Is this an area of strength for your child, or are those strengths being developed?
- What does he want to do differently than you, when he is a parent?
- If she could have any three wishes, what would they be? If she could change anything about herself, what would it be? Why does she feel that way?
- What are his current medical diagnoses? What are the results of medical, educational, and psychological evaluations?
- Does she think she is popular or unpopular? Why does she think this way?

But there are other areas of potential need where it's important to know all you can about your child. If your child has had psychological testing, do you have copies of these reports? How about any medical records or evaluations? Can you find all of your child's school report cards and evaluations? How about results from standardized academic tests? Other than ADHD, what diagnoses and special problems does your child have? Do you have documentation of these issues?

How does your child feel about himself? Does he like himself? Does he think he is popular? Unpopular? In between? Does she think she looks OK? What thing does she like best about herself? Least? Who is his best friend? Why does he like that friend? What does she want to be when she grows up? Where will she live? Will she have children? What does he want to do differently than you, when he is a parent? What does he worry about when he thinks of growing up? What does he worry about now? What is the happiest thing that ever happened to him? The saddest? The scariest? All of these areas of knowledge will serve you well when you are in a position to advocate for your child's needs within school and healthcare settings.

Applying Your Knowledge of Needs to Short-, Intermediate-, and Long-Term Objectives

Once you have a good idea of your child's strengths and greatest needs (the starting point on our map), it's time to set some goals and objectives. These are best broken into short-, intermediate-, and long-term time frames. What is it that you most particularly want in the short term? To get your child through the school day without getting urgent phone calls from the teacher or principal? Or for your child to get to or stay at grade level? For your family life to be less chaotic, with less fighting among siblings? How about for the long term? To graduate from college?

These short-, intermediate-, and long-term objectives, unique for each family, should fit with and build on one another, so that the accomplishment of the short-term goals leads step-by-step to achieving the intermediate-term goals, just as the intermediate-term goals point in the direction of accomplishing the longer term goals. In the same way, when thinking through whether a particular short-term objective is all that important, asking whether it really is a necessary part of achieving an intermediate- or long-term goal can help you prioritize your various goals and objectives.

Short-Term Objectives

Your short-term goals should be those that you can really hope to achieve in the next month or two. These might be as simple as getting your child out of the house and to school on time on a regular basis; setting up a shared homework plan of action, agreed on by your child, the child's teacher, and yourself; taking steps to get the school to set up a school study team staff meeting about your child's needs; learning who are the most ADHD-knowledgeable doctors in your area; or helping your child make and find a friend in the neighborhood. In the box, note that sometimes a short-term objective is something done directly for or with your child, like working

---

Examples of Short-Term Objectives

- Set up homework plan with teacher.
- Get child to school on time.
- Set up reward program for after-school behavior.
- Identify child's potential interests/hobbies.
- Obtain information on local ADHD school programs, talk with other parents using them. Child to complete daily homework by 9 P.M. this month.
- Read basic book on ADHD for parents.
- Attend ADHD parent support group.
- Help child identify list of rewards to work for.

---

with him to identify potential rewards he would want to work for—a necessary step in putting together a behavior therapy program— and other times it will be something that you would do yourself, as a part of obtaining appropriate medical expertise for your child (e.g., getting names of local ADHD-knowledgeable physicians).

Short-term objectives are often specific steps that must be accomplished to achieve intermediate-term objectives. Thus, as a parent, you might set short-term objectives to (1) read up on newly available medications; (2) attend a parent support group and discuss the medications with other parents who have had experience with them; (3) speak with the doctor about it and, if appropriate, begin the new medication. All of these short-term steps and goals may then lead to what you have identified as an intermediate-term goal, namely, *finding a medication with fewer side effects for your child*. Sometimes one short-term goal might be pursued by a parent, while another component is pursued by the child or a teacher, all of which then combine to achieve an intermediate-term objective. Thus, the intermediate-term objective of "Johnny regularly completing and turning in his homework" might be accomplished by several shorter term goals, such as "parent, child, and teacher meet to set up an agreed-on homework plan," "parent and child meet to identify daily and weekly rewards to be used when Johnny completes homework each day and each week," and "parent to follow up by reviewing homework at end of each day."

When you get stuck on achieving some objective, such as just forgetting to do it or finding the goal too difficult, one of the common problems I find is that the goal is too complex and needs to be broken into smaller steps. My daughter finished a 2,000-mile hike recently, from the California–Mexico border to the Canada–Washington border. She found that she could get bored, but she broke up each day into several-hour increments, putting a snack at the end of each period. She didn't think of the 2,000 miles ahead or behind her; she just thought of the much fewer steps she had to take from one snack stop to the next. For ADHD also, as parents, we are on a long journey that is best done in small steps, one step at a time. For example, if your child is flunking most of her classes because she *never* completes her homework and ends up failing most tests, she's not going to transform herself into an A student overnight, no matter how effective her new medication proves to be or how diligent you are in using behavior management techniques. Try to consider what would be definite, attainable small successes, such as completing her homework three out of five nights a week by the end of this month or establishing a study routine starting with fifteen minutes a night for the week before a test, and moving to thirty minutes and then an hour over certain designated intervals over the next few months. If you find that you set but do not reach a goal, try setting fewer or smaller goals. Regularly meeting the goal is much more important than its size. Overly ambitious goals are not good for you, your child, or your long-term staying power on this path you have begun.

Intermediate-Term Objectives

Intermediate-term goals are those that might be achieved over a somewhat longer time period, such as the course of a summer, a semester, or a school year. Such goals might include passing a grade, making a new friend and keeping the relationship going, getting the child tested and into an acceptable special education placement, or identifying the optimal medication strategy for your child. Again, some of these might be activities directly accomplished by the child, perhaps with the parent's assistance; in other instances, they may represent activities that are accomplished by you, your child's teachers, or the healthcare treatment staff.

Sometimes our goals are too lofty. We might say, "I want my child to be on her reading grade level by the end of the year," but if we do not break that goal into small steps, such as *meeting with the child's teacher, reading to the child nightly,* and so on, we run the risk of failing to meet our goals and set ourselves and our child up for disappointment. One good example of this principle occurred when I was working with a young boy with ADHD who had a bad habit of cursing. He cursed often, and after his parents counted how many times, we established that it was up to twenty times daily. I helped the parents start him on a new behavior reward program.

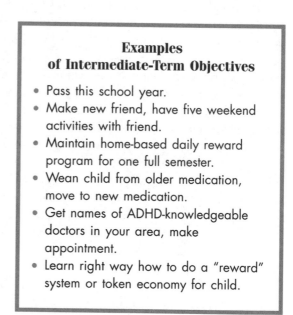

**Examples
of Intermediate-Term Objectives**

- Pass this school year.
- Make new friend, have five weekend activities with friend.
- Maintain home-based daily reward program for one full semester.
- Wean child from older medication, move to new medication.
- Get names of ADHD-knowledgeable doctors in your area, make appointment.
- Learn right way how to do a "reward" system or token economy for child.

Our immediate goal during the first week was to reduce his cursing to fifteen times per day. Imagine how surprised the parents were to learn that we were setting up a program to reward the child for cursing "only" fifteen times daily! Yet asking the child to go cold turkey would have set him up for failure, whereas he could gradually reduce the cursing on a weekly basis, simultaneously earning rewards. It was through this means that his cursing behavior was eventually brought under control, which was our intermediate-term objective.

Long-Term Objectives

Long-term goals are also needed. Where do you want your child to end up? If you could imagine your child ten or fifteen years from now, what would he be doing? Would he have finished high school? Perhaps have a diploma from a trade school? Would she be in college? Holding down a job? Full time or part time? Married, or with a stable partner? Would she have children—your grandchildren? Would he be happy? What are the most important factors contributing to his happiness? Between now and then, what areas of growth do you especially want to see in your child?

> **Examples of Long-Term Objectives**
>
> - Finish high school.
> - Find a career or job that he enjoys.
> - Have long-term friends and friendships.
> - Stay away from drugs.
> - Keep out of prison.
> - Be happily married or with a caring intimate partner.
> - Have feelings of competence and skills at which he is really good.
> - Become a good parent.

All of these "gleams in your eye" are your long-term objectives. But here's the rub: *Your* objectives may not be the same as your child/teenager's objectives, and whether you like it or not, kids do grow up with a mind all their own. So while *your* long-term objectives must be thought about, planned, and hoped for as your child gets older, your objectives must increasingly take into account your child's dreams and wishes, which will eventually hold greater sway than yours . . . as it should be.

But don't despair. What research has shown us is that when parents and youth have good relationships, despite all the challenges of growing up plus having ADHD to boot, youth value their parents' esteem and love, and because of this, they will do many things that they think will please their parents. Not only for the sake of pleasing them, mind you, but because they have taken on and assimilated their parents' values and ambitions, often making them their own. This is true *generally*, though not specifically: Just because you always hoped your child would be a lawyer, and even if you have a terrific and close relationship, don't count out his or her becoming an attorney—or a landscape architect, or an artist, or a salesperson. Be happy; it could have been homelessness or prison! So what might be some reasonable longer term objectives that you would wish for your child? A few are listed in the box. Some of these, such as "stay out of prison," might seem like setting one's sights too low, but remember, every child is different. If we are to fully accept the abilities and disabilities that our children come equipped with, staying out of prison may be a very reasonable, even difficult goal. I once had the pleasure of meeting two parents for whom this was the goal. Once they realized the extent of their child's difficulties with ADHD and had worked through their own sense of loss, however, this was a very good goal for their son—a son they cherished and loved. And because they accepted him so thoroughly, my own sense is that he'll likely do much better, though only time will tell.

Identifying What You Need to Accomplish Your Objectives: What Personal and Family Resources Are Needed, and What Do You Have to Work With?

In forming a plan, we need to keep in mind that, first and foremost, a workable plan is developed by identifying achievable goals based on our knowledge of what resources are needed and what resources are available, followed by setting priorities about which of the various objectives is most important and achievable given the available resources.

Goals and plans must be based on a good understanding of the resources *you* have to work with. Are you ready to tackle the objectives at this point, or are you overwhelmed with other problems yourself? It makes little sense to set out to build a house, only to find halfway through that you don't have enough lumber. Or that you don't have enough help to get the job done. Much better to have built a smaller house! So before we begin to tackle the specifics of forming a plan for your child, let's review our available resources, and identify what knowledge and resources we need ahead of time to maximize our chances for success. What needs to be in place before we can proceed? As parents, there are several questions that we must ask ourselves if we are ready to form a plan and are prepared to take charge. At the beginning of this chapter, I compared forming a plan to getting ready to take a trip from Seattle to Syracuse. So let's first talk about the driver of the car, you.

What Do You Know about Yourself?

"Know thyself," or at least so Plutarch said in *Inscription at the Delphic Oracle*. Even if this is in fact 2,000-year-old advice, it applies today. You must know your own natural strengths and resources. What are the best things about you as a parent? What are your greatest weaknesses? If you have more than one child, what are your greatest strengths with your child with ADHD versus the other child(ren)? What are your own greatest personal challenges with your youngster with ADHD? Is it your temper or frustration tolerance? Is it the ability to find time to spend with him? Is it being able to enjoy her? Whatever they may be, are these challenges the same or different from those of the other children? If it seems to you that all of your weaknesses are with your child with ADHD, and all your strengths are with your other child(ren), then some greater self-knowledge is in order. For example, early on in working with my son with ADHD, I often found myself angry and frustrated with him, and very patient and sweet with my other son. It almost seemed to me that, as parents, we had spawned both a devil and an angel. How could this be? It took a while, but eventually I saw how my own personal feelings prevented me from seeing many of my son's positive traits and caused me to overlook the problems with my other son. It was only when I discovered this that my son with ADHD and I began to turn the corner in our personal relationship, and his anger and oppositionality toward me subsided. The irony in all of this is that I used to feel that my younger son and I were temperamentally most alike, but now I realize that my son with ADHD and I have most in common. This is a source of some amusement to all of the kids, to my wife, and to me.

Over time, knowing myself has included knowing Suzy (my spouse) better as well. Eventually, we began to see how our individual strengths might be used to offset the other's weaknesses. For example, Suzy was an only child, and as she was growing up, she spent long hours in one-on-one time with her very patient father. She seemed to have picked up

> ### Personal and Family Resource Issues to Consider
>
> - What do you know about yourself?
> - Where are you right now? How urgently do you need to make changes for your child?
> - How confident are you that you know what your child needs?
> - What do you feel *you* can handle right now?
> - Do you have the tools, knowledge, and resources to tackle the problems you've targeted?
> - How much help and support might you need from family, friends, and others in implementing your plan?
> - What do you know about your family?

a lot of the same temperament and from the start was exceptionally patient with each of our children. One-on-one she was terrific. For me, being the third of eight children left a different legacy. While I might have been less than understanding or at least "off the mark" in certain one-on-one and other interpersonal situations (particularly with my son), I was very good with working with our five children as a group—"crowd control," as we call it in our family, including family tasks, games, and other activities.

Our kids now have picked up on some level of self- and family-awareness as well. So they like to tell us as parents, "Dad's strict but fun, and Mom's nice but boring." This is said in good humor, but the fact of the matter is that we have learned how to compensate and adjust for each other's strengths and weaknesses. We both know it, our kids know it, and everyone is OK with it. And the upshot of it is, I am a lot more patient and better in one-on-one situations than I used to be. Suzy's gotten quite a bit better at crowd control as well, and has developed a lively set of fun activities that she pursues with each of the children.

In the same way, one parent may be very comfortable helping a child with homework but feel shy about trying to establish friendships for her child, because she's embarrassed at the impression her son has made on other parents in the past; her husband, in contrast, doesn't find this a problem, but tends to get too impatient and critical when trying to help the child with homework. Or one parent might get tongue-tied trying to talk to teachers, school administrators, and doctors but compose great letters and be very organized in writing, whereas the other parent might be quite effective and appropriately assertive in one-on-one sessions with teachers, doctors, and others. Or another parent, who may have boundless patience with her child on the weekends but is almost guaranteed to "lose it" with the kid after work on weekdays, has a spouse with complementary strengths. Knowing such things about yourself, your spouse, other family members should alter the plans/goals you set. You might tackle some area where you are strong and delegate some responsibilities to other family members or professionals. Or you might simply let a certain goal go for now, until you can marshal the necessary resources at another time.

Where Are You Right Now?
How Urgently Do You Need to Make Changes for Your Child?

What is exactly motivating you to make changes right at this point? Are you in the midst of one of your own personal good times, when planning often can be most effective, or are you under siege and desperate to try almost anything? If the former, lucky you. If the latter, it may be some small comfort to know that this is the natural state of affairs. Parents, with or without a child with ADHD, are almost always in over their heads, whether they recognize it or not. But if you are feeling very stressed out at this point, remember that such times are not good periods in which to make major decisions. Your child's ADHD is not going anywhere. Neither are her problems. You have several years to work on solutions, and most solutions for these types of problems do take time and patience.

This parent probably shouldn't have tried to make changes at the time she describes:

> "Frankly, I was overwhelmed. I was working full-time, trying to hang on to my first really good job, but getting angry calls from her teacher on a regular basis. I dreaded coming home and picking up the voice messages. Almost daily, one of them was from the teacher. At one point, after a particularly bad week where my supervisor made a stink about my unpredictably taking time off work, and there were three calls from the teacher—all of them expecting me to 'do something'—I felt there was no way out. That's when I hit bottom. I wanted to crawl away and die. But I couldn't go through with it. It's like childbirth. . . . I almost forget and then can't believe how bad off I was."

The only urgent problems, the ones you must do something about *now*, are those that are physically threatening to your child's and your own health and immediate safety. Otherwise, what may look like a good solution during a point of crisis will often be seen as impulsive after the storm has settled. For most of us, critical judgments and decisions should not be made during such periods. If you are unsure about steps you are planning, or if they are being made during a time of crisis, step back, get away from the problem a bit, and talk to trusted friends or your doctor, minister, priest, or rabbi. Don't just get one point of view; get as many as you can. This is not the time to go it alone.

How Confident Are You That You Know Right Now What Your Child Needs?

Sometimes you might feel uncertain about which are the "right" steps to take to address your child's problems. You might get all kinds of information, some that is contradictory or doesn't really seem to apply to your situation. You may be unclear as to what you should do, much like the parent who told me:

> "I am getting all kinds of well-meaning advice from my family. My sister also has a child with ADHD, but her situation is not at all like mine. Her son Jeffrey is in a really good school, and financially, they don't have anything to worry about. Jeffrey's getting therapy, and he's responded pretty well to medication. But my son Robbie's teacher seems to be on his case, and it is not at all clear whether I should give him medication. The principal seems to be defensive about the teacher, and changing classrooms is going to be an uphill battle. And I can't quit my job and take time off to work all this out. And would it make any difference if I did?"

In my view, this parent is asking all the right questions of herself and her particular situation. Your child has many needs, not only today's needs, but also needs in the near future and even farther down the road. She is likely to have some needs that no one yet realizes. The "right" thing to do is not usually instantly obvious and it becomes clearer only as we try out various things to respond to our children's needs. So it is important *not* to be too cocksure confident here. I don't think any of us can be fully knowledgeable of all of our children's needs, and if we are paying attention, each of us should be frequently surprised by our children (both positive and negative!). This means that you need to look for opportunities to talk with your child about his needs. Even children in early grade school can articulate their opinions about their likes and dislikes, what makes them happy versus sad, or how they would like to handle a given problem. In working with my own son and his bullying of his younger siblings, I found it often helpful to ask him for his views of the problems, what he felt might help him work though them, and so forth.

Your child's teachers and doctors are also be excellent sources of information here, because they have seen many children and have had the opportunity to discover for themselves how various children's needs unfold. No child is the same, of course, and no child's course is perfectly predictable. But the experience of seeing many children grow often gives teachers and doctors an important and unique perspective on what your child's needs might be.

What Do You Feel You Can Handle Right Now?

When your child's problems seem to have mounted up to an intolerable level, you may feel that the only option you have is to fix everything at once, right now. But circumstances can make that impossible, as with this family:

> "There were a lot of other things going on our life at that time. Our other son, Thomas, had been knocked off his bike by a car. He was hanging on by a thread for two weeks. Then there were months of rehabilitation, repeated doctors' visits, piles of bills, you name it. We knew he—Travis, our son with ADHD— needed help and that something was wrong. At first, we thought it was prob-

lems because of his brother's accident. Later, when his brother was more stable, we got Travis his own evaluation. And then we realized he had problems even in preschool. But we were able to work around it then, so it didn't really grab our attention like it does now. But now we can deal with it, too."

Before you embark on some grand plan, ask yourself, does it make best sense for you to attack one urgent problem or lay out a long-range plan? Should you address a simple problem or tackle a complex issue? Handling short-term, more immediate problems can boost your sense of confidence that you can begin to solve these problems. Tackling too much at once will lead to discouragement, frustration, and "learned helplessness." Much better to take small steps and succeed at them than to set goals that are too ambitious. "One day at a time," although a slogan from Alcoholics Anonymous, certainly applies to parents who try to solve all of their children's problems in one master stroke and Herculean effort.

Do You Have the Tools, Knowledge, and Resources Needed to Tackle the Problems You've Targeted?

Don't start on a long journey if you can't see how you will resupply yourself en route. How much do you know about ADHD? Are you confident in your child's diagnosis? Are you confident in your tasks and responsibilities? How should the family deal with your child's problems? Do you have a good handle on what factors *cause* ADHD and know how to differentiate them from those that make its management more difficult but don't really cause it? Or if you are tackling a school-related problem, do you know about your child's educational rights? Or what your child's school resources are? If you are tackling problems related to your child's medication, have you read up on the medication and its effects? Do you know the medication name and dose? Its possible side effects? Do you know where you can go to get this information? If you are feeling overwhelmed and as if you are going it alone, do you know other parents who could provide some encouragement and support? If not, do you know how you can find such parents or support? If you are concerned about your child's doctor, do you know what to expect from your doctor and what to say if you are not getting what you think you should? Do you know what the role of therapy is in working with your child's ADHD? Or how "behavioral therapy" differs from other, traditional forms of psychotherapy? Do you know who is competent to provide various forms of therapy in your area, or at least where to go to find this out?

How Much Help and Support Might You Need from Family, Friends, Teachers, and/or Professionals? And Can You Identify Any Major Obstacles or Restrictions on Your Ability to Plan and to Carry Out Your Plan?

The rest of this book helps you develop the skills you need to offset any deficits you identify and find resources you can tap to fill in gaps in your knowledge.

Before you jump in, trying to fix things, it is essential to know what obstacles you are likely to encounter. You need to have an overview of what lies ahead and what is likely to get in the way of achieving your objectives. Mapping out the obstacles will allow you to determine where you most need to prepare and what supports you need to gather around you before starting. For many parents, perhaps the major obstacle is their own personal doubts and uncertainties. Self-blame is the rule rather than the exception. And when present, it creates uncertainty and doubt at every step. If this applies to you (and it usually does at least in part), do you have someone you can confide in, someone you trust, who can take an objective view (and probably a more compassionate one as well) of the situation?

Other major obstacles lie *somewhat* outside your control, and this must be anticipated. If your child's school situation is very difficult, and few resources or supports are available there, can you counter balance this lack of resources with additional support from family or friends? Or with solid knowledge about how one goes about getting the most from a school system? Do you know other parents who have wrestled with the same issues in your child's school? Certainly, you're not the first, even if you don't know (yet) those parents who may have paved the way before you.

Psychologically, are you feeling on top of things? Do you have enough time and energy to tackle the problems at this point? Or would a frontal assault on these problems strain you or the family's current resources at this point in time? Can the challenges be divided up, so that it doesn't feel like everything is falling on your shoulders? With your spouse? Older siblings? Your own parents? Having others you can depend on will come in handy, again and again.

What Do You Know about Your Family?

In the same way that we must know ourselves and our spouses, awareness of the family's natural strengths and resources is invaluable. If you have other children, how do they feel about your child's ADHD? What do they know about it? Do they have particular areas of strength that can help the child with ADHD? For example, are they good at sports, and can they model or teach this to a younger sibling? Do they have a good relationship, so that they can be friends or talk together? Sometimes, when a child is having a bad day, talking to a sibling can be very helpful. Some siblings even learn to follow their parents' cue in adopting various strategies, such as distraction, to deal with the difficult behavior of a brother or sister with ADHD. Or if Mom and Dad blow their stack at one child, that child's being able to commiserate with the other child can help blow off steam and defuse the situation. Older siblings might be helpful in looking after a younger child with ADHD, giving the parents a much needed break from time to time. This can work as well with an older child with ADHD and a younger sibling. If the relationships are good, an child with ADHD may take pride in some responsibilities or opportunities to look after a younger sibling.

But family members' presence can work both ways, of course. Do they feel there are certain unfairnesses in how they are treated versus how the child with ADHD is treated? Do they misunderstand the situation and just think the other child "always gets his way"? ADHD can add new twists to sibling rivalry that challenge all your parenting resources.

How about your parents, siblings, and in-laws? Are they supportive of your role and your decisions about your child? Are you being second-guessed or criticized for "drugging" your child, or for not somehow being an adequate parent? One parent said, "Some family members and friends tend to think I'm taking the 'easy way out' with regard to medicating my son." Another related: "Coming from a large family (which includes some educators) and having older parents that believe in the stigma of 'mental illness,' some were very uneasy about our son's diagnosis, feeling that ADHD is an 'easy way out' of controlling our child, and/or simply overdiagnosed." In both of these cases, the parents made it part of their intermediate-term plan to inform the uninformed, so that people who were important to them always understood that they were doing their best for their child: "I've made it my personal mission to educate whomever I can educate so that they are made very aware of how knowledgeable we are on the matter, and that I'm working with some of the best docs in the world and going with the most current medical information available, to give my son the best possible chance at a healthy, productive and fruitful life." In this way, they minimized relatives' disapproval of their son and blame aimed at them as parents, which can only sap families of the energy they need to deal with ADHD. Their longer term plans included a goal to spend most of their time with those who were receptive to this new perspective and supportive: "We've had several discussions about our son's care, to the point where we have changed the minds of some, and those that will support us do so. I've learned to disregard most opinions, and have come to rely on a few tried and true friends that now better understand ADHD."

Supportive family members in the extended family can be of enormous value to you if you have them: Spending special time with an uncle, aunt, or grandparent, if planned carefully and done so that the experience is successful for all parties, can be something the child greatly looks forward to and can give you a much needed break from time to time. In our own family, the children had a special time to spend with their grandma and grandpa (my in-laws), with two children rotating into position to visit them each summer. My in-laws were most greatly taxed by our son with ADHD, but because they had him for only a week or two every other year, they were able to keep their sense of being "ADHD-grandson-challenged" under sufficient control that he always loved going there. Eventually, as he matured, they even began to look forward to it! As you might expect, as parents we liked the break, too. (Other ideas for how you can know what to expect from your extended family and friends and strategize to keep your ADHD-afflicted child in good stead with the clan are in Chapter 8.)

Setting Priorities: Which Are the Most Important Objectives? What Are Your Child's Areas of Greatest Need?

Now that we have surveyed the needs, strengths, and resources of the various parties involved, it's time to put them in context, that is, to identify the areas of greatest need. Your child's needs cannot be fully separated from your needs or those of the family's. They interact. Desperate needs in one sphere may override moderate needs in another. As a general rule, a child's needs will increase if the parents' needs are not met, because a child depends on his parents for nurturance and daily emotional support. This is true for all children, but particularly those with ADHD: The child's needs may be even more sensitive to these stresses, with the child less able to bide her time than children without ADHD. But how about you as the parent? Your needs must be met too. Does it make a difference if your in-laws think you are way off base or are critical of your decisions pertaining to your child? What difference will it make if your employer is not supportive? Or if your insurance is inadequate, or you can't find a doctor with whom you are comfortable? Or if the school has few resources or little willingness to assist your child?

Your child has needs outside of those that can be met by you and by the school as well. What if there are no other children his age in the neighborhood? What if the neighborhood is unsafe or riddled with drugs? What if there are not good recreational or sports activities in the area? In the figure below, I illustrate a way to think about how all these influences affect each other and penetrate to different levels. But the figure, for simplicity's sake, can be misleading. How? Well, you know well that not only do parents affect children but children also affect their parents. A child's bad mood after school certainly affects the parent's mood in turn. A child's friends or lack thereof will certainly affect a child's mood. A child's mood or behavior may make him liked or disliked by his friends. And so on. So given all these areas of potential problems and strengths, how do you decide which area to tackle first? Should you tackle problems, and if so, your child's or your family's problems? If my spouse is unsupportive and my child is doing poorly in school, should one problem

Multilevel Influences on Children and Families

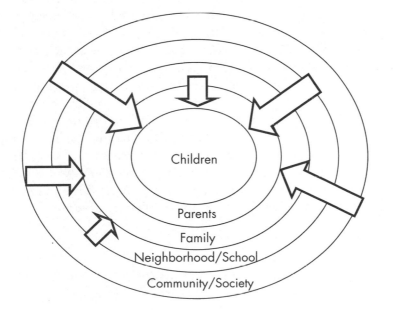

Children

Parents

Family

Neighborhood/School

Community/Society

take precedence over another? Or should I work on increasing strengths and assets first, such as helping my child develop a talent or find a friend, before tackling a problem such as his perpetually not doing his homework? There is no set rule here, but the best rule of thumb I offer is that it is almost always important to work on positive areas for growth simultaneously when you work on "problems." Julie Andrews said it best in her role as Mary Poppins: "A spoonful of sugar helps the medicine go down." When children are always in trouble, it is hard to feel good about themselves, and negative feelings about themselves increase negative behaviors—much like a self-fulfilling prophecy. Our children, like all of us, need to have some areas of their life where they can feel good about themselves, capable, talented, liked, or accepted. So, in my view, always make sure that you combine both.

Guidelines for Setting Objectives and Establishing Priorities

To help you determine what should be the top priorities for getting the best care for your child, let's apply a few simple principles to give you a good head start on figuring out your own version of "first things first."

Make sure your own physical and mental health are sound before you proceed. Said another way by flight attendants, "For those of you traveling with small children, put on your own mask first, secure it in place, and then put on your child's mask." This is rule number one, and the airlines know what they are talking about. If you don't survive the day, week, month, or year, you won't be around to help your child. So if you are barely keeping your head above water, first take time to get help for yourself.

How can you know whether getting help for yourself should come first? Several examples come to mind: First, if you are *severely depressed or in emotional turmoil* yourself, even if you think it is because of your child's difficulties, you need to get enough help to be able to calm yourself down or perk yourself up. There are many effective treatments for depression and anxiety nowadays. Medications known as the SSRIs (selective serotonin reuptake inhibitors), such as Prozac and Zoloft, are quite effective for most folks with anxiety or depression. And they work, with relatively few side effects (or at least minor and temporary side effects) in most cases. There are several effective forms of psychotherapy as well. You should get advice from your doctor about what might be the best course for you, whether a medication, a form of therapy, or both. As one parent put it: "I finally realized that the stresses I was under were now affecting Justin, when he told me he was afraid something bad was going to happen to me. At first this was hard to face, but when the therapist told me that taking care of myself was just another way of caring for Justin, it really hit home. And it was a whole lot easier to deal with him once I began to feel better. He stopped worrying and began to do better at school."

Safety First

Obviously, if there is any significant risk of physical violence or potential for injury, you'll have to address that immediately. Domestic violence, such as spousal abuse or the threat of possible physical injury to your child from behavioral impulsivity (running in front of cars, dangerous climbing behavior, or other risk taking, etc.), or abuse of the child in any form, whether physical or sexual, is an emergency. Ideally, talk to your doctor about these problems. If that is too difficult a first step, talk to a friend, a minister or rabbi, or someone else you can trust.

Attend to Family Problems

Another significant problem that may require immediate attention might be one or both parents' alcohol or substance abuse problems. Like depression, this can endanger your own physical health, and may create great worries in your child and undermine even your very best efforts in many circumstances. For a child to grow and progress, it is most essential that his environment be safe and predictable, and that these core issues not add an additional burden of worry or distraction to the child.

Positive Relationships with Your Child Are Key

While you may put many problems on your to-do list, put this one up close to the top, perhaps the very top. For your child to take advantage of all of the good assistance you are pulling together for him, it will come to naught if your child does not know *and feel* loved by you, the most important person(s) in his life. Don't count on him or her to just come out and tell you this. You have to read the clues by his behavior. Does he like to be with you? Does she want to do things with you? Is she able to talk with you and confide when feeling bad, or when something important to her has gone wrong? If your times with your child are mostly times of tension or conflict, this is an important problem in and of itself, above and beyond your child's ADHD, since research has shown that this is one of the best predictors of poor long-term outcomes.

This is especially hard with a child with ADHD, of course, and being the parent of a child with ADHD is a bit like a double whammy: Not only do you get all the normal challenges that children typically offer to parents, but you also get much more than the normal dose. For us as parents, this makes being patient even more difficult and an even greater virtue when we do! Regardless, finding a way to keep our own feelings of frustration in check is a top priority. If you find you are under too much pressure trying to get all that you can for your child, take a step back: Your family's, your child's, and your own emotional equilibrium need to stay on an even keel.

Final Goal-Setting Points and Principles to Remember

Before you begin to create your specific plan and prioritize objectives within your plan, here are several more principles to keep in mind.

- *First, goals should be flexible*. You must remember that planning is a continuing process and must take into account new facts, new opportunities, and new obstacles.

Don't be afraid to change your goals if you and/or your child are butting heads, either with each other or with outside obstacles. For example, if your child refuses to comply with homework goals you have set up, an alternative goal might be to seek consultation from a therapist. Or if your goal is to get your child some additional school supports, but you can't get an appointment in a timely fashion, an alternative goal might be to write a letter to the principal about the problem, copying other critical parties in the letter (see Chapter 6 for more details on these kinds of approaches).

• *Second, your goals should take the nature of your child's ADHD into account.* Early on, it is tempting to set grandiose goals. But small successes, one by one, are key and are much better than big failures for your child's self-esteem and your own sense of accomplishment. And remember, as you and your child gain success in meeting these goals, you can always set new, grander ones. So if you are exhausted or discouraged, set fewer or easier goals.

• *Third, don't put all your efforts on behalf of your child into one basket.* If you are consuming a lot of energy on one major problem, step back, reconsider devoting some of that energy to a problem where you can see some positive results sooner.

• *Fourth, remember that you are in this for the long run, so if the process of working on your goals does not lead to greater acceptance and understanding of yourself and your child, take a step back, reflect, and reconsider your goals, your progress, your pace, and your available resources.* If things look gloomy, take a break. Then, if things still seem problematic, change one or more of these: your goals, your pace, your expectations for progress, or your resources.

Some Potential Child and Family Needs

Social–emotional needs

- Good self-esteem
- One or more friends
- An area of skill
- Ability to along with others

Medical needs

- Effective medication without side effects
- Available, competent doctor
- Therapist for behavioral therapy

Educational needs

- Teacher(s) that the child likes and that like the child
- Staff's awareness of the needs of children with ADHD
- Availability of appropriate accommodations, IEPs, 504 plans, etc. (see Chapter 6)
- Motivation to do school work, ability to do homework in evening despite ADHD problems

Parent and family needs

- Ability to have fun, play together
- Reasonable sibling relationships
- Parental teamwork to address the child's ADHD
- Absence of major home conflict

Identifying Your Child's Specific Needs

In the chart below, list what you think are your child's and family's most important short-term or immediate needs, categorizing them as shown. To give you ideas about what I mean by needs, I have provided a list of "Joey's" needs to get you started on pages 51–52, grouped in the same four categories.

Don't spend more than twenty minutes on this; just let the ideas flow. Once you have done that, go ahead and see if you can assign a priority to them, starting with the first priority, then the second, and so on. I've given you space for up to four needs per category, but don't try to use them all, if that doesn't make sense to you. To make sure you get specific enough, think about your child's needs from the perspective of *areas in which your child's needs are currently going unfilled*. You might find it easiest to think about the *problems* that your child is experiencing. From that perspective, if a child has low self-esteem, the problem would be termed "low self-esteem" and the need would be for "higher self-esteem." So you can list a need either as the problem the child is experiencing or as what he might need to get over that problem.

Social–emotional needs

_____

_____

_____

_____

Medical needs

_____

_____

_____

_____

Educational needs

_____

_____

_____

_____

Parent–family needs

_____

_____

_____

_____

Creating Your Plan

Now it's time to match your goals—your child's needs that you want to address—with the necessary resources to get the job done. To return to our car and driver analogy, you are the driver, but you also need a car, and sufficient food and fuel to start off. You will also want to identify where you will get additional supplies en route and where food and fuel stations are located along the way. Also, on this trip, who are the people on whom you will rely, perhaps sharing the driving from time to time? So, as any good infantry sergeant would say, this is where the rubber meets the road: putting it all together by prioritizing objectives (or the *needs* that you want to address), then identifying the *specific steps/actions* needed to achieve each goal, along with figuring out exactly *who* will do it, *when*, *with what*, and *how*. Putting this information together transforms your general ideas, concerns, and long-term objectives into a *strategic plan*, with time tables, resources, and so forth, with the short- and intermediate-term goals now becoming *action plans*.

Below I have outlined an example of an action plan based on short-term goals and objectives (and *needs*) for a not-so-unusual child with ADHD. First, let me describe the child briefly. For this plan, identifying information has been changed to ensure privacy.

Example of a Short-Term Action Plan

Nine-year-old Joey has always had a knack for making any calm home situation into a difficult and tense interaction: His apparent jealousy of his younger sister, his constant need to be the center of attention, and his irritation when things seem "too boring" have always challenged and frustrated his parents. It was only recently, after his third-grade teacher raised concerns about Joey's difficulties in learning despite being "a bright boy," and always seeming like he had "a chip on his shoulder," that his parents took him to get an evaluation by his pediatrician. During the interview with the doctor, his parents noted that similar problems with Joey's learning had been raised in first and second grade, but previous teachers thought it was a "maturity problem." After obtaining a medical and family history, doing a physical examination and blood tests to rule out medical problems, and getting behavior problem checklists from Joey's second- and third-grade teachers, the doctor diagnosed ADHD and recommended that Joey be treated with a stimulant medication. After some discussion and disagreement between the mother and father about whether this was a good idea," Joey's father gave in and reluctantly agreed to medication. The pediatrician began methylphenidate five milligrams three times daily. Over the next four weeks, the teacher noted that Joey was "not perfect but a lot better," though he still had problems with peer relations. Joey's relationship with his sister improved minimally, and he still complained frequently that "It's not fair!" His appetite dropped significantly, and he now had trouble sleeping. How might we consider some of Joey's needs from a short-term action plan perspective?

SHORT-TERM ACTION PLAN FOR JOEY

Your child's needs	Approaches <u>Approaches</u> How will the need(s) be addressed? Resources?	Who will do it? <u>Who will do it?</u> Who else will assist and be on your child's team?	When? <u>When?</u> What is the time frame for accomplishing specific tasks?	Outcomes <u>Outcomes</u> Short-term goals and objectives
Social–emotional needs				
Low self-esteem	Help him find a skill; father–son time together exploring sports hobbies	Father and Joey	Start this Saturday	Increased interest in a hobby that he seems to like
Few friends	Discuss, brainstorm with teacher	Mother, teacher	Next parent–teacher conference (two weeks)	Arrange a weekend activity with a classmate
Medical needs				
Is dose adequate?	Discuss with doctor, teacher	Mother, teacher, doctor	Discuss with teacher prior to doctor's visit	Optimal medication strategy that results in few or no side effects; school performance to his ability level
Side effects	Read up, learn about side effects	Mother, father, doctor	Go to CHADD website, read prior to doctor's visit; consider dose or medication change	

(cont.)

51

SHORT-TERM ACTION PLAN FOR JOEY (cont.)

Educational needs

Not performing to ability at school; also, homework not being turned in	Discuss with teacher, get her ideas	Mother, teacher	Call teacher this Friday	Set up long-term plan for Joey's improvement
Problems doing homework in evening	Discuss with Joey, make homework plan he agrees on	Father, Joey	During the weekend father–son sports hobby activity	Happier homework time for all!
	Determine best medication dose	Doctor, mother, father	Next doctor visit	Find better medication or better dose, as above

Parent–family needs

Sibling rivalry	Star chart/reward program chart for "getting along and not teasing"	Parents, Joey, and sister	Start in one week, after family "powwow," where it will be discussed	Decreased conflict between Joey and sister
Parents disagree about medication use	Parents agree to read additional material, discuss it with doctor	Mother, father, doctor	Next doctor visit	Agreement on medication use, communicating same to Joey
Mother feels stressed out in dealing with Joey	Dad to take Joey for chunk of time on weekend	Father	Starts this weekend	Mother feeling less stressed

Now let's try it for you: Take the needs you identified earlier and fill them in on a copy of the blank short-term action plan in Appendix F (p. 252), putting them in each category within their level of highest priority and urgency. Don't worry about intermediate- or long-term plans yet; we'll do that later. You'll find it is quite a bit easier once you get good at creating short-term action plans. Don't be surprised if you can't fill in all of the boxes, because that is what this book is all about: helping you to better identify your child and family needs, identify resources, and map out your strategies to get those necessary resources and approaches to your child and family. As you read Chapters 5–9 you will find the help you need to fill in the missing boxes.

Take another look at your plan and make sure it's as complete as you can make it. From this point forward, we will refer back to this plan, using it all along the way to guide our steps. In addition, to the extent that you can now identify holes in the plan—boxes that you cannot fill in or are unsure about, such as resources, persons, approaches, or even needs—you need to know *now* that these are areas where you need to focus your energies. In essence, your goal from this point forward must be to identify what should go into all of the missing or skimpy areas in your plan, put those steps into place, and execute your plan. That is what you want to get out of the rest of this book, and how you should measure your progress and the extent to which you have become truly "empowered."*

---

*As an aside, if you find this planning process challenging and it is hard to get started, let me encourage you to find and attend a local parent support group, such as CHADD, the National Alliance for the Mentally Ill (NAMI), the Federation of Families (see Chapter 4). Other parents who have "been there, seen it, and done it" will have lots of experience in this. So for starters, make that the first step in your plan!

Four

WHAT YOU NEED TO GET STARTED

Essential Tools and Resources for the Expert Parent

"Talk to other parents. In talking to other parents, find out how their kids are turning out. When you find someone whose child seems to be doing fairly well, ask questions. What are they doing? How are they doing it? Who are the professionals they trust? You get a lot of great information about what to do."

"CHADD has made the biggest difference over time. I have learned a great deal about resources to help my child and other families and it all ultimately came from CHADD or a doctor or psychologist. 1-2-3 Magic saved my sanity and my child's when he was younger, and Ross Greene's Explosive Child *book saved our lives when my child was 12. CHADD's help in all areas has been fantastic. Knowing that it is a developmental disability has been extremely helpful."*

"I ran into a parent on my son's baseball team who was telling me about her son's problems, and we began to share ideas. Later I hooked with up our local chapter of CHADD, which helped a lot. What has made all the difference for me is learning what other parents know, and knowing that I am not alone. It's too hard to try to do this all on your own."

Having a plan, even if only a preliminary one, is an important step forward. But no plan will work unless you have the tools and materials to turn it into action. This chapter lays out all the essential resources you're likely to need, from sources of reliable information, to files and log books for recording your child's progress, to important contacts and groups that can offer support. Additional specifics on addresses, websites, and other contact information are in Appendices B, C, and D; this chapter is intended to give you an idea of what you will need in general and how to use it. This is the substance that will end up filling the "Approaches" and "Who Will Do It?" columns in your action plan. Note also that, as you draw on these resources, you may in fact identify additional needs for your child.

Sources of Information

I've never heard a clearer statement of why it's important to be well informed about ADHD than this message from a parent: "You have to know all you can so you feel comfortable in making decisions that will impact the outcome of your child's life. People are always questioning and second-guessing your decisions. You have to know what you are talking about to feel good about your choices in treatment." Becoming something of an expert in ADHD, then, is not an elective; it's a prerequisite, if you're going to get the most you can from the system for your child. Before you even begin to explore the many available sources of information, however, it's critical that you learn how to distinguish valid facts and figures from opinion, advertising, and simple nonsense.

With so much available nowadays on the Web, it is pretty easy to find just about every opinion under the sun, as well opinions from other solar systems. Sometimes it's easy to tell which ones are downright bizarre and can be discarded instantly, but other times, sensible-sounding offerings prove not to be based in sound science. To put it bluntly, as one parent did: "Be careful in choosing whom to believe! Just because you hear it on the radio or see it in the newspaper doesn't make information about ADHD correct. Parents need to know that Rush Limbaugh, Dr. Laura, and others don't have a clue."

Identifying Alien Notions (the Truly Bizarre Ones)

First, the easy category: those opinions and ideas from other solar systems. As you would expect, these are true aliens. They don't make sense to most people. They may be sensational, however, and even make interesting news, perhaps debates on CNN or other major networks. Remember that an alien opinion, particularly if it is given air time, is just like a foreign object in the human body that stimulates an immune response. So, too, alien notions will generate strong reactions among those persons from more respected, more earth-bound persuasions. So very often, if you see two parties in a public media debate, lots of heat may be generated, plenty of arguments will be made. But remember, most media outlets, sometimes even supposed news media, succeed only if they attract listeners, viewers, and readers. An argument between supposed experts about a hot topic is sure to be more entertaining and to sell more copy than a single, dry presenter or presentation. Here are a few signals that what you're about to hear is an opinion from Mars:

• *"There's a conspiracy."* First, the alien opinion is a bit more likely to be based on some version of a conspiracy theory. There are many iterations of the conspiracy notion, as applied to ADHD. It is an easy target: "The drug companies and the psychiatrists are in cahoots, just trying to line their pockets, and at your child's expense!" Or "Even the federal government is on it!" And how about this one? "The scientists are faking their data, just to get papers published and to get more grants." OK, time for common sense: If the president of the United States couldn't get away with covering up a break-in, or even a clandestine relationship, how could thousands of doctors, hundreds of scientists, many federal bureaucrats, and dozens of drug companies get away with a true conspiracy against children all across the United States, even the world? Think of the thousands of eager young reporters who would love to make their careers by exposing this most monstrous of all cover-ups!

• *"No one is telling you the truth but me"* (also known as the *"We will never lie to you"* approach). This one you should be able to see coming, once you have a good handle on the conspiracy theory. With almost everyone else involved in the conspiracy, there aren't too many folks left, are there? Therefore, conspiracy theory types tend to be pretty lonely. And because aliens are usually easily spotted by most humans, they often have to resort to other means to generate support. They may have to prey on others who are vulnerable, perhaps other like-minded conspiracy theorists, those who are disenfranchised.

• *"Write your Congressman and put a stop to this!"* Long-distance methods, such as reliance on simple, media-based techniques of persuasion, write-in campaigns, and so forth, are a good means to avoid being spotted as an alien. Hitler was an alien, albeit a very persuasive one. It might have been hard to detect what he was up to by simply attending his staged media events. For aliens, close-ups are not good, and prolonged one-on-one conversations will usually blow their cover. Dealing with the day-to-day realities of how to help one's child with ADHD is not easy for one with an alien mind-set.

Instead, aliens prefer to stick with media appearances, inflammatory websites, or encouraging you to write your representative, all clever ways to drum up interest, even belief and support, from others! And it works more often than we might like to believe. For example, in my experience, if you look around, you can almost always find a few among our many fine national and state representatives who might be susceptible to misinformation and glad to get some C-SPAN airtime promoting it, as if tilting at windmills!

Beware! But remember, you don't have to get on the spaceship to detect an alien. Instead, talk with knowledgeable other persons. Gather more facts. Be skeptical of what you might see and hear on television, without further verification and reading the original sources.

For example, let's say you hear on some television program that medication causes brain damage in children with ADHD (actually, this is a pretty common one you are likely to encounter). First, get the reporter's source. Was it initially reported and published in a highly respected scientific journal, such as *Nature, Science,* the *Journal of the American Medical Association,* or the *New England Journal of Medicine?* Fully credible and reliable journals have independent scientists review each potential publication before it is allowed to see the light of day. Alien pseudoscience *never* passes this hurdle. If the reporter doesn't cite his source, e-mail the station and request the name of the scientist who published the paper, as well as the journal name, title of the article, volume number, page numbers, and date of publication. If it was-n't published, and/or if it wasn't done by a researcher at a respected university, you can probably stop right there; you have plenty of things to do with your time other than chase down every alien notion. If it was published, look it up based on the au-thor/scientist's name, or e-mail/write the author to ask for a "reprint," with full de-tails on the article (journal and article names, date, volume and page numbers, etc; I'll tell you how to do this later). Alternatively, or in addition, discuss it with your doctor and see what he or she says.

Another strategy is to avoid using television altogether as your source of medi-cal information; that's usually where the alien notions especially flourish. They also do well as short blurbs in newspapers or when picked up by some columnist. Instead, read credible, nonsensational magazines or information put out by the federal gov-ernment or nonprofit organizations through their websites. Good (but not infalli-ble) examples include *Time*, *Newsweek*, and *U.S. News & World Report*. Credible websites include those sponsored by the National Institute of Mental Health (NIMH, *www.nimh.nih.gov*), the Center for Mental Health Services (CMHS, *www.mentalhealth.org*), the Food and Drug Administration (FDA, *www.fda.gov*), and nonprofit parent support organizations such as CHADD (*www.chadd.org*) or NAMI (*www.nami.org*). Another good bet is the highly respected and accurate in-formation printed in the weekly health sections of respected newspapers such as the *New York Times* or the *Washington Post*. In all these examples, the information is *al-most always* well researched and accurate. And when you encounter conflicting in-formation from reliable sources, start over, check the sources, and read more. Talk with other parents who have a child with ADHD, and who have been at it for half a dozen years or so. If you get caught up in the conspiracy theory, remember that doc-tors, folks working in drug companies, and bureaucrats have children, grandchil-dren, nephews and nieces, too, just like you and me. Would they do such terrible things to their own relatives?

Let's further track the "medication causes brain damage" idea as a good example of an alien notion. Well, in fact, there was a report almost two decades ago by a re-spected group of researchers in an acceptable (but not top-notch) journal on what is called a "retrospective case–control study," comparing twenty-seven adults with a history of childhood hyperactivity and twenty-seven adult control subjects, using computerized tomographic (CT) brain scans. Findings showed evidence of *cortical atrophy*, or possible loss of brain tissue in the outmost layer of the brain, the cerebral cortex.* Case–control studies such as this one are an important part of science, but are considered to be at one of the lower levels of scientific evidence, since they in-volve only the comparative description of a group of cases with normal controls. Cause and effect cannot be determined, but such reports are important, because they alert scientists to areas where better-controlled, prospective, but more-difficult-to-conduct studies might be needed. So despite the fact that millions of people have been treated with ADHD medications as children, with tens of thousands of them

---

*Nasrallah, H. A., Loney, J., Olson, S. C., et al. (1986). Cortical atrophy in young adults with a history of hyperactivity in childhood. *Psychiatry Research, 17,* 241–246.

having later brain scans for various reasons (such as head trauma), this finding has never been reported since. But it is still easy for any alien to pick up this one report, cite it as proof of a cause-and-effect relationship between persons' history of medication use and abnormal brain scans, and claim that it applies to all children. Given the weight of all of the other evidence (i.e., no reports of such findings among doctors always eager to publish any dramatic finding), a much more likely explanation for this one finding would be some other factor (e.g., chronic alcoholism, or even ADHD itself, regardless of treatment).

So let's finish the story: Just this last year, scientists from the NIMH (the leading scientific body in the world in mental health research) reported in the *Journal of the American Medical Association*, one of the world's top medical journals, that they had scanned children repeatedly over a period of years, comparing 152 children with ADHD treated and not treated with medication with 139 age- and sex-matched children without any history of ADHD or stimulant medication treatment. Their results? The brains of children with ADHD treated with medication were slightly *larger* than those of untreated children with ADHD! And compared to the normal control group, children with ADHD showing the greatest evidence of smaller cerebral tissue brain volumes were those with *no* history of medication use (5.9 percent smaller than the age- and sex-matched control subjects). Also of note was their finding among all children with ADHD that reduced brain size was related to the severity of ADHD symptoms, indicating that the differences in brain tissue volume are related to ADHD, not to its treatment.

So note the clues that should help you sort this one out: It was a large study, almost 300 children, with carefully chosen control groups; it was current (instead of decades old); it used the latest technologies (MRI, or magnetic resonance imaging, instead of the much less precise and now out-of-date CT methods); it studied children prospectively and longitudinally (not a retrospective case–control study or a single-case report); it was funded by the federal government; and it was conducted by topflight researchers at a respected research institution (vs. someone who maybe can cite only having been formerly affiliated or loosely affiliated with such an institution). The other interesting thing you will find out if you look up the earlier article by Nasrallah and colleagues is that these authors, being respected scientists and not aliens, were very cautious in interpreting their findings, noting that the results could be due to ADHD itself *or* to its treatment, and they advocated the importance of additional studies. And in fact, now over a dozen subsequent studies have been done, showing that children with ADHD have slightly smaller brain sizes (five to seven percent) than children without ADHD. A report by Castellanos and colleagues is the latest in this series and provides the most definitive evidence to date that these differences are related not to treatment but to ADHD itself.*

*Castellanos, F. X., Lee, P. P., Sharp, W., Jeffries, N. O., Greenstein, D. K., Clasen, L. S., Blumenthal, J. D., James, R. S., Ebens, C. L., Walter, J. M., Zijdenbos, A., Evans, A. C., Giedd, J. N., & Rapoport, J. L. (2002). Developmental trajectories of brain volume abnormalities in children and adolescents with attention-deficit/hyperactivity disorder. *Journal of the American Medical Association, 288,* 1740–1748.

Identifying Flaky Notions: Separating Sense from Nonsense

Flaky opinions are qualitatively different from the bizarre or alien ones. Flaky ones don't usually have strong, seemingly credible spokespersons. Instead, they are faddish, they tend to come and go, and they don't get nearly so much media attention. Examples might be the notions that the cure for ADHD is blue-green algae or a good course of chiropractic manipulation. These ideas seem surprising, catch you or others off guard, and for most people lead to a skeptical set of follow-up questions, or at least a look of surprise and politely raised eyebrows. The ideas, usually at the outset, don't make sense.

The Taxicab Driver Test

If you are unsure, try the taxicab driver test: Next time you are in a taxi, tell the driver about the notion or theory and see what he thinks. Or if you don't use taxis, ask your hairdresser or barber. Find out if she would be willing to spend money on it. If she thinks it's flaky, it probably—but not always—is. Now, don't make the mistake of asking what she thinks the truth or the real facts are. She is just as susceptible to media misinformation as the next person; she is just as likely to have her own pet theories as the next person. So while the back of a cab is a pretty good place to get advice from someone who is good at spotting scams, it is not the place to get the facts. Like you, the driver or hairdresser is going to have to do some reading to know the facts.

Checking with Your Child's Doctor

This is an opportunity to check with your child's doctor. For starters, you might ask, "What do you think of the recent report about . . . ?" If the answer isn't crystal clear, a follow-up question may be needed: "So you think there's nothing to this? Why?" But remember, the doctor's input may be helpful, but it is not necessarily definitive or authoritative. How might you know if he is "on the money"? This can be difficult, but one rule of thumb that might be helpful is how specifically he answers. The more specifically he answers, the more likely it may be that his opinion is sound. So if he brings up a specific objection (e.g., "It's interesting, but since it's the first and only study of its kind, I think it's too soon to give it any credence—certainly too early to change our approach to treating Johnny on the basis of it"), you can get a good amount of additional information. If, on the other hand, he's not specific but just expresses an undefined skepticism, perhaps his opinion isn't well founded; maybe, he's embarrassed that he hasn't even heard the report and doesn't want to appear ignorant. Or just maybe too busy? Here, you'll have to use your best judgment and do some additional study on your own. But one who says he hasn't read the report in *Time* magazine when you know that *Time* cited the leading pediatric journal in its article might tell you something about how much time this doctor spends on his own continuing education. The most problematic response is that of the doctor who gets defensive or appears offended by your inquiry: This does not re-flect the basis of a good parent–provider partnership, something you are definitely going to need.

Identifying Seemingly Sensible but Unproven or Incorrect Notions

From here on out, it gets a bit tougher (but well within your ability), because you can't readily tell a seemingly sensible but incorrect idea from a truly correct idea from a distance, or without doing some homework. Also, seemingly sensible ideas sometimes have not yet been well researched, so it is unclear whether they are cor-rect. And when more studies are done, some turn out to be correct. So seemingly sensible ideas need to treated with caution: Reserve judgment if they haven't yet been studied. Be skeptical but open: some will pan out, though many will not.

The list of proposed causes of ADHD that fall into the category of sensible but unproven ideas currently is actually fairly long: the impact of food additives (for some but clearly not the majority of children); stress and trauma; environmental toxins; lack of necessary early environmental experiences that encourage the devel-opment of attention control and motor behavior; lack of critical minerals or vita-mins in the diet; environmental deprivation/neglect; prolonged early exposure to highly stimulating, perhaps overstimulating environments (e.g., video games, televi-sion, particularly in the absence of other appropriate experiences); and so forth. For treatments, the list is somewhat shorter: biofeedback, rhythm (metronome) therapy, special elimination diets, use of food supplements, various experimental therapies (holding therapy, etc.).

Identifying Sound Scientific Information

This is where you have to get up close to the problems and to the best sources of in-formation. While the Web is a good place to get lots of information, it doesn't dis-criminate good from bad. You must. Fortunately, many other parents have formed organizations to gather and screen information, separating sense from nonsense and then making that information available in user-friendly formats. Examples of such organizations of parents are CHADD (Children, Adolescents, and Adults with ADHD; *www.chadd.org*), Federation of Families for Children's Mental Health (*www.ffcmh.org*), the National Mental Health Association (*www.nmha.org*), and NAMI (National Alliance of the Mentally Ill, *www.nami.org*); more information is available on all of them in Appendix B. All of these organizations share several characteristics (see sidebar).

In contrast, organizations to beware of have these characteristics: They purport to have the "true" answer, often a single solution. They make money for themselves. Often, they may have a tool or technique to sell. They usually have no scientific ad-visory board. Or if they do have a board, the "scientists" do not have a strong history of publications in respected, peer-reviewed scientific journals, nor do they have a consistent track record of receiving carefully scrutinized taxpayer monies to gener-ate solid scientific information. Look out for the organizations whose claim to fame

---

Characteristics of Credible Organizations

1. These organizations have stood the test of time. They have been around for a long time, usually because they provide a service (including support and accurate information) that others have valued enough to pay dues and/or contribute their own personal, volunteer time.
2. They have a democratic structure, with elected officers at local, regional, and national levels. In order words, they attempt to be responsible and responsive to their members. Bad apples usually get weeded out over time. Or, as stated in the Sermon on the Mount, "By their fruits ye shall know them."
3. They have a scientific advisory board consisting of volunteer scientists, who provide advice to members in screening sensible from nonsensical information, science from pseudoscience.
4. They are nonprofit. They provide lots of no- or low-cost assistance and information to other parents. Why? Because help was there for them when they needed it for their children.
5. They are centered around and shaped or run by the true experts in the trenches: parents much like you, who differ perhaps only because they have "been there, seen it, done it, and gotten the T-shirt." They have lots of experience in raising their own children with similar problems and, often public spirited, they want to make sure that other parents don't have to go through what they went through: years of misinformation, uncertainty, and unnecessary suffering for their children and their families.
6. Because of all of these characteristics, which make them credible, they often receive grants, paid for by *your* tax dollars, to reach out to other parents to disseminate accurate information.

---

is the endorsement of one or more movie stars, a few dramatic testimonials of a small handful of parents, dramatic cures, and conspiracy theories.

Given the importance of separating fact from fiction, to give you a head start, I've listed on the next page a few of the more common myths and "myth-conceptions." Please note, these myths are actually fairly common and are held not only by conspiracy theorists but also sometimes even by responsible parties, such as news commentators, physicians, friends, and relatives.

Types of Information

There are many ways to get good information, and you may want to tap any and all of them, depending on what works best for you, your lifestyle, your timetable, your preferred means of learning. These include books, websites, information prepared by associations and organizations, professional journals, parent magazines, conferences/lectures/workshops, videos, and even direct word-of-mouth from other parents. Any

Myths versus Facts about ADHD

Myth: ADHD is overdiagnosed and overtreated.

Fact: Each year, only about one-half of the children with ADHD across the country receive any treatment. While there may be regional pockets of overdiagnosis, the bigger problem nationally is underrecognition and underdiagnosis.

Myth: ADHD is caused by crowded classrooms and poor parenting.

Fact: ADHD causes are rooted in brain functioning, with well-demonstrated differences between healthy children and children with ADHD. While stressful home and school environments can be *distracting* to any child, they do not cause ADHD.

Myth: Children grow out of ADHD, so adolescents and adults don't need treatment.

Fact: Two-thirds of children with ADHD will go on to have significant continuing symptoms as adolescents, and up to one-half will still have these problems as adults. Treatments work just as well for adolescents and adults as they do for children.

Myth: Medication is only marginally effective in children with ADHD.

Fact: Stimulant medication has been proven extremely effective in the treatment of children with ADHD.

Myth: Medications don't help in the long run.

Fact: Recent studies show that children treated with medication and careful monitoring continue to benefit from medication treatment, even after periods up to three years in carefully controlled studies. Longer term studies also indicate benefits into young adulthood.

Myth: Medications are harmful to development.

Fact: Medications have been extremely well tested by the FDA and found to be both safe and effective. Neuroimaging studies show no negative effects on brain development. And longer term growth studies indicate no significant problems, except possible small effects on height and weight. These effects may be due to *delays* in growth rather than actually smaller eventual size. Longer term follow-up studies indicate that children with ADHD attain their expected height and weight, based on their parents' height and weight.

Myth: Girls can't have ADHD.

Fact: Girls have fewer hyperactive symptoms and conduct problems than boys. Because they often have the inattentive subtype of ADHD, they are often missed or diagnosed later than boys. The ratio of boys to girls with ADHD is about four to one. By young adulthood, the ratio is more equal, perhaps even one to one.

Myth: Children with ADHD are not eligible for special education.
Fact: If impairment in school functioning exists because of ADHD, children are eligible for special educational services.

of these learning methods can suffice all by itself, since there is a lot of good information out there.

So don't overwhelm yourself and think you have to do it all, to catch every fact, to read up on every possible scrap of information. You can't, and trying to do so will exhaust you and lead to a point of diminishing returns. So how do you know when you have enough information? Simply stated, when all the columns and rows in your plan are filled in, and when each of the strategies appears to be working. Just another reason to keep that plan at your elbow, particularly as you're getting started. Eventually your plan will be second nature, and you'll be getting and using information by instinct.

Books

Like this one, books can be a handy way to get lots of good information consolidated in a single place. But remember, books should be treated cautiously. Many times, a book may be full of good information but have lots of other stuff you don't need. Any book might include good information and bad information, all nestled side by side in its pages, making it quite challenging to separate fact from fiction. Simply relying on a well-known publisher or book company is not sufficient, because, in the long run, what generates book sales is what leads a book to get published, not the quality or accuracy of its contents. Look for books published, written, or endorsed by some of the leading parent organizations listed earlier.

Some books are designed more for what is called the "trade" press, that is, information prepared for consumers, edited to ensure user-friendly language. Fact and fiction alike get published here, but if you have identified a good reputable source (a respected parent or government organization, well-recognized and credible doctors and/or scientists), you will find lots of quite readable information here. But not always. Lots of personal opinion, and even some misinformation, may have wormed its way between the book's covers. In contrast, there are professional or scientific books, usually put out by a select group of publishers that target professional groups. These books are often "edited volumes," with one or more scientific editors (usually an MD or PhD) and lots of individual scientists and doctors writing individual chapters. These publishers are intent on ensuring that the information is solid and will often submit the book to independent review before it is published. At the end of the book or each chapter, you will find lots of references to scientific publications, because the chapter's content should be based on a scholarly review of accepted facts. Although such books can be good sources of information, they can be difficult to read and often may still reflect the final opinion of one scientist whose opinion and scientific judgment may not always represent the state of science.

I have provided a more extensive list of books that may be useful in Appendix E. These titles were chosen through my knowledge of the authors' scientific reputation and past works, my personal review of the book for its scientific integrity, or both. New books are always coming out, so if you want to determine the potential usefulness of such a book, you can employ a strategy similar to mine by looking up the author's name in PubMed, the National Library of Medicine's (NLM) search service that provides at no cost access to over eleven million citations via the Internet (*www.ncbi.nlm.nih.gov/pubmed*). Simply type in the book author's last name followed by the first and middle initials (e.g., Jensen PS, Nasrallah HA, or Castellanos FX). If you find a bunch of citations in the NLM database by that person on ADHD and related topics, you can be sure that she is quite expert, since all of her listed articles had to pass through that scientific review process before publication. But remember, most books do not go through the same scientific review process as a published scientific journal article, so even if the author is expert, you may still be getting some personal opinions mixed in with facts—just another reason for becoming your own expert! Another tip you can use is to examine the book jacket and look up the names of the scientists recommending the book: Are they also expert?

This is not a perfect strategy, however, because many professionals write books for the general public and are not necessarily scientists. Instead, they may focus on translating scientific findings into helpful common language for use by parents and others. Nonetheless, even many of these will have research experts recommending the book on the book jacket or in the preface, and so forth. Always ask other parents what books they've found useful and why. This can save you lots of time (and expense) on books that prove not to have exactly what you're looking for. Books that parents have told me they found useful in various areas include Edward Hallowell's *Driven to Distraction*, Russell Barkley's *Taking Charge of ADHD*, *ADHD and Teens* by Colleen Alexander-Roberts and Paul T. Elliott, *Boundaries* by Henry Cloud and John Townsend, *ADHD and Driving: A Guide for Parents of Teens with ADHD* by J. Marlene Snyder, *From Chaos to Calm* by Janet E. Heininger et al., Ross Greene's *The Explosive Child*, and *1-2-3 Magic* by Thomas W. Phelan.

Websites

The Web is a convenient, easy, and very fast way to get lots (sometimes too much?) of information right away. If you are looking for a single fact, entering a few critical search terms into a credible website's search engine can be very effective. For example, government organizations, such as the NIMH, the FDA, and the CMHS, all mentioned earlier, will often have the results of recent studies summarized somewhere on their websites, and each of these agencies allows you to use their own search engine to search its website. Sometimes you can use a more general search engine to find facts anywhere in the millions of sites across the entire World Wide Web.

One very effective search engine is *www.google.com*. If you go to this site, for example, and enter terms such as *methylphenidate* and *side effects*, with each phrase separated by the word *and* (i.e., "methylphenidate and side effects"), you can find almost every possible fact and fiction about the side effects of the most commonly prescribed medication, methylphenidate (better known by its various brand names, e.g., Ritalin, Concerta, Metadate). Another Web search service is called Copernic (*www.copernic.com*). This service requires you to download some software (the "basic" version of the software is free), and it also does an excellent job, drawing on many other search engines, then organizing and prioritizing the results. Although both work quite well, the problem with these and most other search engines is that they don't review the quality or accuracy of the content they find for you, so you have to go back and rely on guidelines like the ones presented earlier for identifying accurate sources of information. Remember, there are lots of aliens out there, and they all have websites, too. Web information sites and sources ending with *.gov* or *.org* tend to be more consistently reliable than those ending with *.com*, which often are trying to sell something, including *misinformation*. *Caveat emptor*—"Let the buyer beware."

But even nonprofit organizations and websites can be misleading, such as sites with attractive names such as "Center for Science in the Public Interest" (*www.cspinet.org*), which has a highly publicized but misleading report and advice on the supposed links between ADHD and allergies. (This organization actually does excellent work in nutrition. So even an organization that does good things isn't necessarily going to be infallible in all areas. This also happens pretty frequently to scientists who render opinions in areas where they are not expert.) In contrast, the search engine PubMed (described earlier), supported by the federal government's NLM, searches only well-respected scientific publication sources and journals. Medical journals don't get put into its search engine unless they meet specific standards for scientific quality. For this reason, it won't search for information in sources such as *Time* or *Newsweek*, because these magazines are not scientific journals, even though they will from time to time have good scientific information content. But they may also publish seemingly sensible but incorrect notions and sometimes even alien notions. Remember, the stories and interpretations of scientific findings in such magazines have been filtered through the writer/reporter's eyes, understanding, and personal biases, as well as through those of the editors.

Newspapers and Magazines: News You Can Use?

Here, you also have to be careful. What sells this type of print media is "news," both fictional and factual. Your local respected newspaper and national magazines are chockfull of both kinds. There are several important exceptions, however. The *Washington Post*, the *New York Times*, and the *Chicago Tribune* all have excellent weekly health sections written by full-time science writers trained in translating science information into user-friendly language, separating nonsense from nonsense. Their sections are also overseen by editors, who, with the assistance of full-time "fact checkers," are concerned with getting the facts right and preserving their newspapers' reputations for accurate reporting. These are *usually* excellent sources of information, but only rarely will some aspect of ADHD be covered. Remember, though, even the mighty *New York Times* (aka "the Gray Lady") faced an extremely embarrassing and compromising situation in 2003, when it was learned that one of its reporters had simply concocted stories and invented the "facts" to support them. The lesson to be learned here? You have to read everything with a health dose of skepticism.

In contrast to those generally factual and accurate health columns, don't assume that just because an article has an Associated Press (AP), United Press International (UPI), or Reuters News Agency byline it is conveying accurate information. All that these bylines mean is that one of these news syndicates picked up the story from *some writer somewhere* and made it available on the newswire for any paper to reprint. Any given newspaper may pay a fee for this service, so that its staff doesn't have to write everything using its own local reporters. While this saves them time and money, it doesn't spare you the task of separating sense from nonsense. So apart from the exceptions of the high-quality health sections, be on your guard and read between the lines.

Association/Organization-Produced Information

As noted earlier, there are a number of high-quality membership organizations devoted to preparing user-friendly scientifically based information and tools to improve children's ADHD care. The two organizations with ADHD as a strong focus are CHADD (*www.chadd.org*), and ADDA (the Attention Deficit Disorder Association; *www.adda.org*). The CHADD membership tends to consist principally of parents of children and adolescents with ADHD, to some extent adults with ADHD, and a fairly large contingent of treatment providers who work with ADHD families. ADDA is a bit more focused on adults with ADHD. The annual meetings of these organizations are also good places to get good information, although opinions and personal experiences are often a large part of such meetings and may not always reflect good science. In contrast, such organizations' Web pages and written materials tend to be scrutinized and reviewed by the associations' scientific advisory board.

Scientific Journals

The peer-reviewed journals are where scientists report their studies, and where they are scrutinized by others. *Peer-reviewed* means that once a scientific manuscript has been submitted for potential publication, the journal editor sends the manuscript out to volunteer, independent scientific reviewers who provide a careful critique of the manuscript and make recommendations about correcting any potential problems in the study, its interpretation, or the author's claims and conclusions, and so forth. These reviewers may also recommend that the article be rejected for publication. In fact, with the very best journals, only a small proportion of papers are accepted, which means that *usually* only the results of well-described, carefully executed, and highest quality scientific studies ever show up in the scientific journals. This peer-review process ensures that scientific study methods and findings are checked and double-checked by others who have no vested financial interest in the studies' findings. In addition, this careful publication process allows other scientists to come to their own independent conclusions as to whether the results are credible, and whether the study's results should be rechecked by some new team of investigators who repeat the study. By and large, only those scientific findings that have published in respected journals and have been repeatedly replicated by independent teams should be regarded as factual. Remember, anyone—scientist or not—can make a claim, but without this kind of scientific process, the supposed facts may be bogus. For savvy parents, just as for serious scientists, the watchword should be "In God we trust, but from all others, demand data!"

Which journals are the best? In the area of ADHD, the following journals are all excellent and often cover ADHD: *Journal of the American Academy of Child and Adolescent Psychiatry (JAACAP)*, *Journal of Abnormal Child Psychology*, *Journal of Attention Disorders*, *Journal of Child Psychology and Psychiatry*, *Journal of Child and Adolescent Psychopharmacology*. More general journals, such as the *Archives of General Psychiatry*, *Pediatrics*, *American Journal of Psychiatry*, *Biologic Psychiatry* and *Journal of Consulting and Clinical Psychology*, are topflight but have ADHD articles only from time to time. The *Journal of the American Medical Association*, *New England Journal of Medicine*, *British Medical Journal*, *Science*, and *Nature* are all world-class journals, but they rarely publish anything on ADHD. Science-related journals for the lay public include *Scientific American* and *Psychology Today*, which are also usually quite good.

It is a vast area, since there are literally thousands of new articles on ADHD now published each year, so you might feel overwhelmed. Don't be. Remember, there are many other wise people out there like you, also trying to filter this information, including doctors, schools, organizations, and other parents. Don't assume you always have to do it alone. As one parent put it, "Having contacts in the medical community certainly helped . . . but looking in quality places for quality information is the best way to start—CHADD, local/state and national special education associations and parent associations, and the state department of education."

Current Perspectives and Future Research Directions: Diagnosis, Outcome, Cause, and Treatment of ADHD

To keep up with developments in our understanding of ADHD, you'll have to check in with reliable information sources on a regular basis over time. One way to get a broad perspective on recent advances and ongoing areas of investigation is to look at the latest research by browsing through some of the journals mentioned in this chapter or searching the PubMed website (*www.ncbi.nlm.nih. gov*), typing the term *ADHD* into the entry space. To see what research is currently being conducted and

(cont.)

supported by the federal government, but not yet published, go to one of the websites of the NIMH Computer Retrieval of Information on Scientific Projects (CRISP) at *crisp.cit.nih.gov*. Simply click on the box entitled "Go to CRISP Query Form," type in *ADHD* where it asks for a search term, and you will get the project and scientist name and brief descriptions of all currently funded federal research on ADHD.

To give you a head start on current scientifically based perspectives, here is a summary of findings relevant to parents of kids with ADHD, up to date as of late 2003.

Diagnosis

Current Perspectives

- Some sources have suggested that ADHD is on the rise, but we really don't know for certain. Clearly, as it has become better known among parents, providers, and teachers, it is more likely to be diagnosed now than it was twenty years ago. It is possible that it is also on the rise, but no good studies have explored this possibility yet. Other childhood emotional/behavioral disorders such as depression are thought to be on the rise, however, so we cannot rule out the possibility that ADHD is also on the increase.
- Despite claims that it's a fad illness of the last ten or fifteen years alone, ADHD has been around for a long time—with reports of children who appear to have had the syndrome as far back as 100 years ago—and appears in every country in which it has been studied.
- Most studies, including those done by my colleagues and me, indicate that ADHD is often missed. Clearly, there are some cases of overdiagnosis, but the best available studies indicate that although about five percent of children have ADHD, only half of them get diagnosed and treated. Children with ADHD in poverty, as well as in minority communities, are at two times greater risk of being missed.
- The fact that your child's doctor may use a different term for the disorder does not necessarily mean he is behind the field. An earlier version of the American Psychiatric Association's diagnostic manual, DSM-III, called the diagnosis "attention deficit disorder, with or without hyperactivity (i.e., ADD and ADD/H)," and many practitioners simply find these terms more sensible and clearer.
- Scientists no longer believe, as they once did, that girls are overrepresented in the inattentive subtype. Among adults, males and females appear to be equally represented in ADHD, inattentive subtype.
- In Appendix D, I have listed some of the important books on ADHD diagnosis (e.g., DSM-IV published by the American Psychiatric Association), as well as a recent state-of-the art and very comprehensive book that presents all the latest research in one place, up through the end of 2002 (see the edited book by Jensen and Cooper, 2002).

Future Research Directions

- The Centers for Disease Control is conducting studies to explore the possibility that ADHD is on the rise.
- Whether there really are distinct subtypes of ADHD, and how ADHD differs between boys and girls, is still under investigation. When we look at older kids who don't seem to exhibit much hyperactivity or impulsivity, are we seeing kids with the inattentive type of ADHD or those with the combined subtype who are experiencing the natural course of the disorder?
- Studies are actively under way to determine how various children with ADHD differ in terms of specific genes, differences in brain scans, psychological tests, and the like.

Outcome

Current Perspectives

- Research findings suggest that forty to sixty percent of youngsters with ADHD will have this problem during adulthood. And as best we can tell from follow-up studies of children with ADHD now grown up, those who make good use of all of their abilities can succeed just as fully in life as anyone else.
- In the most definitive study to date, the large Multimodal Treatment of ADHD (MTA) study still being done by seven sites across the country (see details below), only one-third of children who were treated with intensive behavior therapy alone achieved normal functioning by the end of fourteen months of treatment, according to parents and teachers. In contrast, two-thirds of those receiving carefully adjusted medication plus behavior therapy achieved normal functioning. Just over half of children receiving only careful medication treatment achieved normal function. The bottom line? All things being equal, most kids are likely to achieve the best outcomes if medication is a part of the overall treatment package. Children with lots of complex problems especially needed the combination of both treatments.

Future Research Directions

- One study on outcome is the largest and most comprehensive longitudinal study of ADHD children to date, the MTA study, with which I am involved. It began with 579 seven- to nine-year-old children, each treated by one of four approaches: (1) standard community treatments (whatever the family wanted and found available in the community); (2) fourteen months of university-provided, best-possible medication treatment; (3) fourteen months of university-provided, intensive behavior therapy; or (4) fourteen months of the combination of both university-provided treatments, and medication and behavior therapy. The MTA study has reported treatment results and outcomes up through two

(cont.)

years, and the federal government is supporting up to ten years of follow-up study, to examine these children's adolescent and young adult outcomes. These findings will provide the most definitive information to date on the outcomes of children and youth with ADHD, determining which factors, including treatment, are associated with optimal long-term outcomes.*

Causes

Current Perspectives

- *Genetics.* Studies have shown that children with a parent or sibling with ADHD are five to eight times more likely to develop this disorder than children with parents or siblings who do not have ADHD. Studies have found that certain forms of specific genes are more likely to exist in children with ADHD than in those without ADHD. The two major findings concern genes related to the brain's chemical signaling functions involving the neurochemical dopamine: the dopamine transporter gene (abbreviated as DAT1) and the dopamine receptor type 4 gene (abbreviated as DRD4). These findings are quite recent, emerging just in the last five to seven years, and are now among the best replicated findings in all of psychiatric genetic studies, child or adult.
- *Pregnancy and birth complications.* Some studies suggest that birth complications, such as prolonged or difficult labor and elevated bilirubin levels (jaundice) during the initial days, occur more frequently in those with ADHD than in those without ADHD. In addition, some factors, such as exposure to tobacco smoke or alcohol during pregnancy, as well as to lead during early childhood, appear to modestly increase the likelihood that a child will develop ADHD. See Appendix D for additional references, particularly a chapter by Swanson and Castellanos in the book by Jensen and Cooper.**
- *Neurological.* A number of studies have shown a correlation between the risk of ADHD and trauma to the central nervous system, such as occurs in a head injury with loss of consciousness. Studies also show differences in the size or structure of portions of the brain (cerebellum, corpus callosum, and caudate nucleus) in those with ADHD.

Future Research Directions

- The big challenge for future studies of the causes of ADHD will be to find a way to determine which causes apply to specific children. As we get better

---

*MTA Cooperative Group. (2004). NIMH multimodal treatment study of ADHD follow-up: 24-month outcomes of treatment strategies for ADHD. *Pediatrics, 113,* 754–761.

**Swanson, J. M., & Castellanos, F. X. (2002). Biological bases of ADHD—Neuroanatomy, genetics, and pathophysiology. In P. S. Jensen & J. R. Cooper (Eds.), *Attention Deficit Hyperactivity Disorder* (pp. 7-1–7-20). Kingston, NJ: Civic Research Institute.

knowledge of patterns of susceptibility genes, this may be possible: Thus, lead exposure or tobacco may only meaningfully affect children with certain types of genes. Or among those with strong family histories of ADHD, we should eventually be able to learn how what kinds of environmental and preventive interventions may be offered to lessen or eliminate the effects of ADHD altogether. What kind of special early environments might be required for the child with a particular set of ADHD genes to develop "work-arounds," so that his brain attentional and motor control systems develop more normally? Given what we already know about the plasticity of the young, developing brain, such possibilities will clearly become realities, just as recent research has shown for children with so-called fixed "learning disabilities" (See footnote for research by Paula Tallal, Michael Merzenich, and colleagues.)

- Genetics is a rapidly advancing area of science, so you may want to refer to the website of the previously mentioned NIH CRISP database at *crisp.cit.nih.gov* to see what kind of studies and potential findings may be waiting in the wings. In the CRISP Query Form, type in *ADHD* and *genetics*. For a nice summary of the research to date, see the chapter by Swanson cited in the book cited by Jensen and Cooper, Appendix D.

Treatment

Current Perspectives

- The ADHD medications have been studied extensively, and no meaningful long-term side effects have been discovered, after forty years of use. There are short-term effects on appetite and sleep, but these usually subside. Intermediate-term effects are noted on height and weight, but these appear to vanish by the time the child reaches late adolescence or adulthood. As best we can tell, the child appears to eventually "catch up" with his peers in terms of height and weight.
- A recent National Institutes of Health (NIH)-funded study found that for children with ADHD and tics, the combination of clonidine and methylphenidate was more effective than either medication alone. Clonidine also seems to benefit some children's impulsivity, and help children who are having trouble falling asleep.
- Many other studies, not just the MTA study, have documented that stimulant medications are the best studied and most effective way to treat ADHD

(cont.)

---

*Merzenich, M. M., Jenkins, W. M., Johnston, P., Schreiner, C., Miller, S. L., & Tallal, P. (1996). Temporal processing deficits of language-learning impaired children ameliorated by training. *Science, 271*, 77–81.

Temple, E., Deutsch, G. K., Poldrack, R. A., Miller, S. L., Tallal, P., Merzenich, M. M., & Gabrieli, J. D. (2003). Neural deficits in children with dyslexia ameliorated by behavioral remediation: Evidence from functional MRI. *Proceeds of the National Academy of Sciences, 100*, 2860–2865.

symptoms. By and large, the stimulants appear to be more effective than other medications such as the tricyclic antidepressants, atomoxetine, or bupropion (even though these other medicine do in fact work), but this is based mostly on careful clinical observations, rather than head-to-head studies comparing the medications to each other. In Appendix D in the book by Jensen and Cooper, the major studies and publications are cited that have established these facts.

- In general, providers agree that if a child's height, weight, and overall development are monitored carefully, the benefits of medication usually outweigh any potential side effects. According to the NIH's 1998 Consensus Statement on the Diagnosis and Treatment of ADHD, the short-term trials of stimulants have provided strong support for the safety and effectiveness of medication treatments for children with ADHD.

- *Alternative treatments.* The term *alternative treatments* or *alternative medicine* usually refers to any treatment other than medication or standard behavioral treatments. A variety of alternative therapies have been proposed and continue to be advocated for the treatment of ADHD, including special diets, fatty acids, vitamin and mineral supplements, herbal remedies, biofeedback, hypnosis, metronomes, and meditation. Generally speaking, most treatment alternatives for ADHD lack systematic research that supports their appropriateness and efficacy. Other interventions, particularly those that are ingested, may cause serious side effects, such as liver damage from overingestion of some minerals (i.e., iron) or vitamins (A, D), neurotoxicity, cardiac arrhythmias (ephedra), and other medical complications. Ineffective treatment of any kind may also significantly delay access to and benefits of effective and appropriate treatment. The single best source on alternative treatments is a chapter by L. Eugene Arnold, also listed in Appendix D in the Jensen and Cooper book.

Future Research Directions

- Naturally, new medications are always being developed and behavior therapies refined. See Appendix D for books on medication and Appendix G for medications commonly prescribed as of the publication of this book. But to keep up to date as new treatments are developed, you might want to check PubMed (*www.ncbi.nlm.nih.gov*) once a year or so, or in the event that your child develops a comorbid condition. Use the search terms *treatment* and the actual name of the condition (e.g., *ADHD* or *depression*), and restrict the search to the last year, so you don't get hammered with too much information. Alternatively, the latest information on all of these disorders is usually the NIMH website and can either be downloaded or ordered by fax to be sent back to you at no cost (*www.nimh.nih.gov*). Likewise, because NAMI is an "all types of mental disorders" organization, you can go to its website and usually get recent and accurate information (*www.nami.org*).

Management Tools to Help You Do Your Job

Accurate information—whether about the cause and treatment of ADHD generally or about your child's personal experience with medication side effects or special education services—is valuable data. You need a way to keep track of it all and preserve it for later reference. The following tools are essentials.

File Cabinet and a Filing System

When your child has just been diagnosed with ADHD, you may believe you can keep track of his care just by filing insurance claims and other papers in the same files you've been using for other family healthcare matters. But in my experience, ADHD has a way of producing quantities of paper that quickly become unmanageable. So I strongly suggest that you acquire some sort of separate file cabinet just for ADHD-related material. Lacking all else, a cardboard carton designated for this sole use will do, but most office supply stores carry inexpensive cabinets or file boxes, many of them equipped with folders, dividers, and labels.

One way to categorize the information might be on the basis of your plan, such as according to your child's particular needs. Many papers, handouts, or articles may be of a general nature, so you will need a general or "unfiled" folder. As you become more expert, some of those articles that seem "general" now may fit into a specific folder later. Some items may seem to fit multiple categories. If so, put that piece of information into the folder that it fits best, and in each of the other related folders, put in a single sheet of paper noting that that piece of information is filed in another folder. Said one parent:

> "I have documented, all in three notebooks, (1) IEP meetings, (2) past mental health facility treatment (all past medical records are in my possession), (3) present medical status (includes medication logs). I also have a notebook divided into different info sections—CHADD, ADDA, Internet sites for ADHD, etc. I subscribe to any ADHD newsletter I can get my hands on as well."

It is a good idea to review your file cabinet every couple of months or so, weeding out outdated information and, when needed, forming new categories based on your evolving interests and understanding. Reviewing the "unfiled" folder is also important, since you may find that you can now identify new categories under which that information can be filed. Be careful not to fall into the "packrat trap," in which it seems like any piece of paper or article is always needed. Too much irrelevant or redundant information can overwhelm your filing system and your human capacities to keep things organized. So weed out what you don't really need. One good rule of thumb is that if you don't access or use that information after one year, it is probably not needed and should be discarded.

Medical Records, Psychological Testing, and Educational Reports

You may be surprised to hear this, but as the person who has the best handle on all of your child's needs, you must have all of your own copies of your child's medical, educational, and testing records. Yes, doctors and therapists have always regarded the medical records as theirs, private, even *sacred*. Speaking from my own perspective as a doctor, the charts, our reports, everything all the way down to our incomprehensible scribbles, have always been part of our very own, special domain. But, increasingly, we doctors (but not all of us yet) are realizing that for the best medical care to take place, patients and families need these records. Why? There are many reasons, each unique to the circumstances of a given child and family. Families move, doctors and other healthcare providers retire, healthcare plans change, other specialists get involved and need the information, and so forth.

In the past, when a doctor or therapist needed the results of a report or test that someone else had done, she would obtain your signed permission and then mail that permission form to the other provider, requesting the records. That person or clinic, with more than enough other things to worry about, would *try* to handle your request—assuming the letter even arrived, the copy machine was working, staff was available to follow up, and they could find the record! Given these blessed circumstances, they would then copy the record and mail it to the provider requesting it—all without your ever seeing it! Truly amazing and bizarre. But in a recent report, the National Academy of Science's Institute of Medicine concluded that the medical record really *belongs to the patient!* Remember, *you* pay the doctor's fees, you hired him or her to perform a service, and by golly, you need to see the product you paid for!

Not every doctor likes this turn of events, mind you, and many will be downright resistant. But the facts remain the same. You need these records, so that they are there at your fingertips when *you* need them for your child, *not* when the doctor or medical system can find the staff, time, and copy machines to make it happen. So don't settle for less.

A simple polite request will often suffice. If a verbal request is insufficient, putting the request in writing might be necessary. Failing that, you have several options: First, discuss it with the doctor and find out what is holding things up. Don't be timid: This is your child, and remember, if it weren't for you and parents like you, the doctor would not have an income. It is your right to have this information. If the doctor seems testy, this is a bad sign: You may not have the best kind of partner you need in getting the best care for your child. And it may be more trouble than it is worth to wring the information out of the doctor. He may not, in fact, be keeping good records and may have little to give you! As a second option, consider upping the ante by sending a second letter, writing at the top "SECOND REQUEST," with a "cc:" at the bottom to some lawyer, such as "Mal L. Practice, Esq." or "I. M. Serious, Esq." You may not have to really retain a lawyer, if you have a family lawyer/friend who will let you use his name. As a third strategy, rarely needed, get the lawyer to write the letter on her stationery. These are the big guns, so don't use them on this problem unless you really need the information in the worst way. There are plenty of other battles to fight, and this may or may not be the most important one.

Managing Your Child's Medication: Tips for Parents

- Know your child's medications.
  - —Learn the trade and generic names of the medications.
  - —Keep a list of the medications in a handy place.
  - —Keep records of the names, dates, dosages, and prescribing doctor of all medications.
  - —Learn the purpose of the medications.

- Know the potential side effects of your child's medication.
  - —Have the doctor list potential side effects.
  - —Notice side effects and report them to your doctor.

- Follow the doctor's advice about a medication.
  - —Make sure your child takes his or her medication only as prescribed.
  - —Find out from your doctor or pharmacist what food or drinks to avoid.
  - —Find out if any activities should be restricted.

- Safety
  - —Don't give any over-the-counter drugs or any other medication without first checking with your doctor.
  - —Keep all medication out of the reach of children.
  - —Have an adult supervise your child's intake of medication.
  - —Never give your child's medication to another person or let your child take a medication not prescribed by the doctor.
  - —Tell your child's other doctors, including dentists, what medications your child is taking.

Also, you don't need every new doctor's note that he makes into the chart for routine follow-up visits: That would be tedious for him, and it would be pretty meaningless for you. But you do want copies of any significant tests or evaluations, laboratory studies, letters, and so forth, as well as a summary of the overall diagnosis and treatment, if you have to change doctors.

Educational records are usually much easier to get. Why? Plenty of lawsuits have established parents' rights to this information, and federal law requires that when schools do testing and make placement determinations for your child, those records must be made available to you. A simple request will usually suffice if the records aren't provided outright. But any or all of the preceding steps can be used if you need another resort.

Your Medication Log Book

Most children with ADHD will at some point be on medication. The array of medications that are now available is dizzying and very hard to keep track of. If your child is placed on medications, it is quite likely that the first dose of the first medication will not be the final medication step. You will need to keep track of this, including the specific name of the medication, the dose in milligrams, the number of times per day that the medication is to be taken, and the date that that medication dose was started. While all of the currently available, most commonly used medications are quite safe, any of them can have temporary, usually mild side effects. These side effects, such as trouble sleeping or irritability, can sometimes get confused with the normal ups and downs of being a child with ADHD, regardless of treatment. The doctor can best tell if a side effect is occurring by noting the time of day the side effect occurred, with respect to the last dose of medication, and the only way he will know this is if you watch for it.

Medications are also switched over the course of growing up, and for us as parents, it often is hard to remember whether our child had in fact been tried on a given medication, what happened in response, and if it wasn't continued, why not. Keeping your own medication log in a three-by-five-inch notebook will prove invaluable and over time will give you, more than anyone else, the best knowledge of the medications' effects on your child.

Insurance Records

The last kind of information you will want to keep track of are records of all your medical bills, claims submitted to insurance companies, amounts paid by the insurance company, and amounts you paid. If you are in a health maintenance organization (HMO), you may be spared many of these headaches, since most of the care you receive inside an HMO is simply provided without any further billing process. But for most of us, that is not the case. In addition to all the records, bills, receipts, and check stubs themselves, you may want to keep a simple log of all expenses that looks something like this:

Date	Type of service, provided by	Total fees	Amount billed to insurance, date filed, by whom	Amount paid by insurance	Amount paid by me, check stub no.

Keeping track of this information serves several purposes: First, you may be able to deduct some of these medical expenses from your income taxes. Second, as often as not, insurance companies and doctors' offices make billing mistakes, and you may get a bill that you or the insurance company already paid. The only way to prevent yourself from overpaying is to keep track of how much you have paid, who paid what, and when. While this seems like a lot to keep track of, in fact, it just takes a minute or so to file things in the right place when you receive them or make a note on the log. It will save you hours and hours later, because you are sure to need this information at some point in the future.

Sources of Support

Support can come in many forms. It might mean that you have someone you can confide in or who can give advice. At other times, it could mean that you have a shoulder to cry on. Research studies have shown that there are two major types of support that people need in stressful circumstances.

Emotional Support

This type of support is the kind that helps you when you are feeling bad about yourself, perhaps when you are feeling like you have failed as a parent, or are feeling guilty for wanting to throttle your child, or feeling overwhelmed that you just can't do it all. This kind of support may be especially important in preventing depression or overwhelming anger in yourself. Depending on your own circumstances, a spouse might be a good source of emotional support. But sometimes a spouse may not fully understand what you are dealing with, which can make the situation even harder to bear. Your spouse may in fact blame you, so not only will you not get much support from this spouse, but she or he will be adding fuel to your emotional fire. Or sometimes you might have another person, perhaps a friend or confidant upon whom you can rely. The most important characteristic of people who can provide optimal emotional support is the ability and willingness to *listen*. They may provide advice, but that is usually not the most helpful thing this kind of support offers, and in fact, if the advice is laced with too many "you shoulds" it may be just what you don't need. One good way to know that this is a good source of support for you is that the person makes you feel understood. As simple as this sounds, it is critical for each and every one of us.

Tangible Support

The second kind of support you often need is very practical: Someone who can help out at a moment's notice by watching your kids when you need to go to handle a problem at your child's school. Someone who is willing to babysit so you can have some time to yourself. Like emotional support, this might come from a spouse, a close friend, or others. It might be a service offered by your church or synagogue community, or it might even be a service you pay for.

Another potential source of tangible support might come in the form of "respite services," special services provided by an agency or human services organization that works with the child, often in some type of recreational format, as a means of giving the parents of a child with a disability some much needed time off. The availability of the services varies widely from area to area, but the best way to find out about such potential resources is to call your city or county department of human services. These agencies go by various names, such as Department of Human Services, Child and Family Services, Disability Services, Mental Health, or perhaps Social Services. You'll have to check around, but if you know any parent with a child with any type of special needs (e.g., not only a child with ADHD but also a wheelchair-bound child or one with autism or Down syndrome, cystic fibrosis, heart disease), she may know of such resources that she draws on for her own child. Also note that many of the same agencies may have access to special or emergency funds set aside to assist a child with medically related needs that are not covered under normal insurance provisions (tutoring, "Big Brother–Big Sister" support). If you don't ask, you won't know. (See also Appendix B for such resources.)

The point is that tangible support is the way we all avoid burnout and get through our day. If we have plenty of emotional support but inadequate tangible, practical support, the emotional support will eventually give way and prove insufficient. Likewise, tangible support without emotional support just won't cut it in the long run. And because you are in this for the long run, make sure you line up both types of support before you desperately need them and have already become overwhelmed.

One parent reported, "I have had a lot of support from our family physician regarding treatment for both our daughters. For example, for the school, I generally write a letter of what I would like done, changed, etc., and he attaches it to his letter, stating that it is his opinion that the idea should be carried out." Still another parent spoke of negative "support," warning: "Don't let anyone make you doubt yourself. Arm yourself with as much information and support as you can. Distance yourself from unsupportive, negative, or uncaring people. Life is hard enough with an ADHD child without a negative support team."

Critical Contacts

A final important resource is those go-to people that can save you countless frustrating hours, whether you're trying to figure out exactly how to appeal a denial of insurance coverage or ironing out a new wrinkle in your child's classroom accommodations. Sometimes these people just present themselves to you, but more often, you have to cultivate them. Almost everyone likes to be helpful, but like you, almost everyone is busy and on the verge of being overwhelmed. To get them to make that extra effort to be helpful takes a bit of extra effort on your part: being pleasant, being nondemanding, making requests in a way that makes others want to meet them, sending special thank-you notes after a service has been done, and so forth. Most parents find it's well worth the time and effort.

The "Answer" Person at the Clinic

Let's say you need a copy of your child's records, and the receptionist is busy. What do you say? As a rule, the best strategy is not to be demanding or angry but to approach that person with a friendly smile, perhaps followed by something like, "I know you must be terribly busy, but I am wondering if you can take a moment to help me." Wait for an answer. Most people will say, "Sure." Why? You have given them the chance to be helpful. You have pointed out that you understand what their day must be like. You have indicated that your request is not too extensive. And if they are too busy, or don't help right away, be understanding. You need this person, so there's no use losing a potential ally. Instead, recruit the receptionist into your ranks by bringing her a hot cup of coffee the next time you're at the clinic, by going out of your way to greet her personally and pleasantly, and so on.

Keep in mind, though, that sometimes you're not going to get anywhere with the person who seems like the obvious choice to fulfill your request. Maybe the receptionist isn't all that efficient, and even though she should be the one to supply copies of files, she just isn't going to do it in a timely fashion, if she does it at all. In that case, you should try to identify someone else in the office who can and will do the job. Maybe you can ask a sympathetic nurse how else you can get the copies you need. Sure, it's not her job, but if you explain your dilemma and say you'd really like some advice about how to get what you need without stepping on any toes, she may very well intercede on your behalf, and this may then be your go-to person at the clinic.

Also keep in mind that you may simply have made false assumptions about who does what at your child's clinic. Maybe the job descriptions don't fall into traditional slots at this particular office. If you feel you're running into a brick wall in trying to get your requests answered, ask the doctor or therapist who does what and whom you should ask—for file copies, referrals, appointments, consultations that don't require the doctor, and so forth.

Your Contact at Your Insurance Company

The same principles apply to other types of critical contacts, such as the person who processes your insurance claims. First, you need the person's name. It is a real person on the other end of the line or letter. But you need to make him real to you, and yourself and your child's needs real to him. In such a situation, finding out who handles your information or your claims is a very good strategy. This will often take place on a phone call, where a simple "I wonder if you can help me, please?" is a good start. Once you have found the right department and get that person's name, you thank him that you have finally been able to reach *someone*. You then explain your dilemma. Listen carefully and try to do all he suggests. When you mail in the information, you might find it a good idea to send him a copy of the claim form, with a special note attached, such as "I can't thank you enough for taking time to talk to me today. I'm the person that told you about my red-headed son who fell out of a tree. So here's the claim form we talked about. I appreciate your helping us out. I'll check back to see if there is anything else needed. Sincerely, Me."

When you end up dissatisfied with the quality of information you receive from the first people you reach by phone at your insurance company's general number, you have the option of asking to speak to a supervisor, but that is certainly likely to alienate the person you're speaking to. Sometimes the best approach is to call back several times, to double-check what you've been told, or to ask for clarification. At most large insurance companies, you'll never get the same person twice. That can be a good thing, though, because eventually you might hit on someone who is empathetic, knowledgeable, and willing (even eager) to help. When you do, make sure you get the person's name and direct number, and don't hesitate to be effusive in your gratitude for having found someone who can really help. We all love to be told we're good at our jobs. Call that person's direct number or, if there is no direct route, ask for the person by name when you call. If you're told she's unavailable or are given some other run-around, state unequivocally that you'll wait to talk to her and insist on knowing when you'll be able to reach her.

Your Contact at School

School contacts are critical. Here, it is important to remember that a school is a small system, a bit like a family. All the teachers know each other. The principal knows all the teachers. At the end of the day, they must all get along, even if they don't get along with you. So here you do not want to make enemies. You will only incite all of the family members to close ranks around one of their own. For example, it is hard for a principal to get down on one of his teachers. In the event of any problem between a parent and teacher, it is the natural instinct for the principal to defend the teacher, unless you are the fifth person that week to complain about that teacher. Much better to befriend a teacher than to do battle with her. All battles have costs, and there will be casualties on both sides, possibly including your child. And unlike other situations, where when push comes to shove you might be able to fire your child's doctor, it is hard to fire a whole school, particularly since school districts have rules about such things as letting children attend schools outside their geographic area.

In some situations, particularly when your child has more than one teacher, you might find that you can form a good relationship with one particular teacher, who can then act as "your friend in court" with other teachers or with the principal, when special arrangements for your child are needed. Alternatively, a school counselor, the school secretary, or the school psychologist—any one or several of them— might prove to be that critical contact who can get you the report you need, the special accommodations, or the ear of the principal. Prior to starting a school year, ask other parents which teachers or counselors seem to be especially supportive of kids who have learning or attentional difficulties.

A Lawyer

The point of finding go-to persons at all the sites where your child needs services for ADHD is to avoid creating adversarial situations, which are rarely the best route to getting what you want. "Win–lose" approaches, as Steven Covey said in the *Seven Habits of Highly Effective People*, where the other party must lose so that you can win something for your child, never work as well as win–win strategies. So sometimes a lawyer is necessary, but involving one should always be a last resort. Only after you have used up all of the other approaches, talked with other parents to make sure there are no tricks you haven't tried, and then searched your soul for anything else you might think of, and only when your child's health and well-being are at stake, should you bring in the big guns. These strategies are often effective if you have se-lected your goals carefully and, as often as not, systems such as schools will often back down, since they don't like such battles. But just remember, winning a battle is not the same thing as winning a war.

It's a good idea to have a lawyer in case you need one, however. Other parents who have used one before for these purposes may be your best guide here about what you have locally available. Ideally, you would want a lawyer who has had experience with children's disability rights and/or has previously successfully challenged school-proffered services. You may have to call several law firms, specifically asking whether the firm has this kind of expertise, and if not, which firm in the area might have such expertise. And when you find one, ask about the firm's experience in this area: How many cases of this type has it handled? Can they give you a few names of satisfied clients? The firm won't do this without first getting the client's permission, but it is worth asking. Anyone who is nondefensive in response to your questions should be willing to do this, and if you find someone like this, go with him or her. See Appendix D for more information on legal resources.

Refining Your Plan

Before we leave this chapter, pull out your short-term plan, and add to it any needs you may have for additional information about your child's medical care, your insur-ance plan, your child's testing and school records, and other related items. Be sure to fill in these needs, as well as how you plan on getting that additional information. In starting to explore information resources, have you found any gaps in your under-standing of ADHD? If so, does that indicate areas where you should develop set ob-jectives to become better informed? For example, if you have learned some new facts about medication or the role of behavior therapy, do you need to set a short-term objective to find a healthcare provider who can offer that type of treatment? Do you need to set a short-term objective to talk with other parents about the providers they know in your locale who might be a good fit for your family? Are there some al-ternative treatments you have been using that you should discuss with your doctor, or perhaps do more research on? On the next page is an example of a short-term plan refined in the medical and educational needs areas.

SHORT-TERM ACTION PLAN

Your child's needs	Approaches How will the need(s) be addressed? Resources?	Who will do it? Who else will assist and be on your child's team?	When? What is the time frame for accomplishing specific tasks?	Outcomes Short-term goals and objectives
Social–emotional needs				
Medical needs				
1. Information on what your insurance covers	Call company, ask health benefits manager at work	My husband	1 week	Accurate information on coverage
2. Previous medical records	Ask doctor for records	Me	Tomorrow	Complete set of records
Educational needs				
1. Previous school testing records	Send letter to school with formal request	Me	Tomorrow	Complete set of school testing results
Parent-family needs				

82

Part II

WHAT TO EXPECT AND HOW TO GET WHAT YOUR CHILD NEEDS

Five

GETTING THE BEST
FROM THE HEALTHCARE SYSTEM

"We were lucky to have a great pediatrician who helped us with Robbie's diagnosis. He helped us with questions, talking with Robbie's teachers, etc. Finding a therapist that seems responsive and knowledgeable seems to be a challenge. We have seen a total of five therapists or counselors. One of them has been great—a licensed social worker. He has been helpful in navigating Robbie's school issues with respect to behavior. However, he is limited to that area of expertise. Robbie is currently under the care of a psychiatrist for his more general issues. We are still determining whether he is meeting Robbie's needs."

"One of the biggest areas we have had issues with is other doctors (e.g., her orthodontist) or teachers. These folks seem to act like it's a nuisance to them rather than understanding that Sherrilin can't help having ADHD. This is a shock, given our expectation that they knew about ADHD and ways to handle it."

"The medical system is one area where we have been most fortunate. I have known my son's pediatrician for fifteen years. He treated my daughter, as well as my son. My son's counselor is a wonderful man—he is also ADHD—and is excellent in relating to the feelings that my son has such a difficult time expressing."

"A big dilemma was getting inconsistent diagnoses. Probably the worst experience with a physician was in fact with one that actually diagnosed my son with ADHD after a ten-minute office visit. He prescribed a huge (forty-milligram) dose of Ritalin to start with. My son was eight at the time. This pediatrician only prescribed this dose for the morning. He then went on to say that the initial adjustment to the medication is pretty 'rough.' Since I was a professional myself and had had some experience working with a physician, I requested that he adjust the medication gradually. I was most concerned that the large dose in the morning with nothing in the afternoon was an invitation to rebound disaster. He reacted as if the suggestion was totally ridiculous and refused to cut down the dose. We changed pediatricians."

In this chapter I discuss an issue that is likely to be one of your central concerns: how to work with doctors, nurses, other healthcare providers, and the insurance system. Many of you will get hung up in this area, because it can feel like you have to repeatedly challenge the system just to get something done on behalf of your children—whether it's getting your doctor to provide a fuller explanation of your child's diagnosis or treatment plan, obtaining the medical records and reports that you need to pass on to your child's school, or getting the insurance coverage your child needs. By and large, we are taught to respect authority, and we tend to cut doctors and other healthcare professionals a lot of slack in terms of what we expect from them and how we handle setbacks when they seem to disappoint us. "The doctor knows best" is what most of us have been taught, implicitly or explicitly. So to challenge the doctor's opinion might suggest we don't trust the person in whose hands we've placed our child's health. To ask too many questions might make us appear stupid.

As if getting the help we need for our children weren't enough to accomplish, finding a way to get through this psychological minefield might seem next to impossible. Difficult, yes. Impossible, no. Necessary? Yes—if we are to become effective case managers and ensure the best healthcare of our children with special medical and educational needs. In this chapter I offer some ideas for handling these difficult situations, starting first with physicians and other medical professionals, then moving on to other parts of the healthcare system, such as insurance and managed care companies.

Making the Doctor Work for You

Remember principle number 4 here: You (or your insurance company, which you pay via premiums) pay the doctor's salary, so in a real sense, she *does* work for you. This does not mean that you should act entitled or take an attitude of "the customer is always right." But in the long run you have to be comfortable with your relationship with your child's doctor; you need to "find a good doctor that you click with," as one parent put it. And since your ultimate goal is to get your child the help he needs, you need to make sure you're getting the help and advice your child should get from the doctor. If not, it's important to work these issues out, seek another opinion, or find another doctor. "You have to take great care in selecting the professionals you need" is the way one parent put it. "Then you need to listen to them and trust them—until you have good reason not to."

As I said in Chapter 2, many of us doctors are not terribly comfortable with the notion that we work for the patient and family. We like to think of ourselves as "professionals," which is shorthand for "I am the expert, so what I say goes, and you should accord me some respect." Respect is all well and good, but it doesn't mean staying mute and meek. If you're having surgery, you're pretty much putting your life in the hands of the surgeon and anesthesiologist, and not much input is required from you. But managing a child's ADHD requires *you* to do most of the surgery per se, making you a critical member of the treatment team. You, the doctor, and others will be involved in a lot of ongoing discussion, problem solving, and sharing of opinions and concerns. You have to find a way to make sure the doctor or therapist is providing everything his profession offers for kids like yours, while knowing where your expertise ends and the practitioner's begins. (Though I use the word *doctor* through much of this chapter, and I'm often referring to the practitioner who can write prescriptions for any medication your child needs, the principles and advice here apply to all of the practitioners listed in the following box.)

Glossary of Practitioner Types

Psychiatrist—a doctor (MD) who specializes in psychiatry, able to treat children and adults with emotional or behavior disorders. Can also prescribe medication.

Child and adolescent psychiatrist—a doctor (MD) who has completed training as a psychiatrist, plus training in treating children with emotional and behavioral disorders. Can prescribe medication and do therapy.

Child psychologist—a psychologist who specializes in children and adolescents. See "Clinical psychologist" below.

Clinical psychologist—a mental health provider with a doctorate, PhD or PsyD, in psychology who tests, evaluates, and treats children and adults with emotional and behavior disorders. This provider cannot prescribe medication.

Clinical social worker—a mental health provider with a master's, MSW, or doctorate (PhD) in social work, who evaluates and treats children and adults with emotional and behavior disorders. Cannot prescribe medication.

EdD—indicates persons with a doctorate in education. They sometimes do psychotherapy.

LCSW—indicates that a person is a *licensed clinical social worker.*

MSW—indicates a master's degree in social work.

MD—indicates that a person has a doctorate in medicine and is able to prescribe medication. This may include **pediatricians, psychiatrists, neurologists,** and **family practitioners.**

Pediatrician—a doctor (MD) who specializes in treating all types of childhood illnesses.

PhD—indicates that a person has a doctoral degree, usually in psychology.

(cont.)

Physician's assistant (PA)—person with special training, less than an MD, but able to treat and prescribe medication under an MD's supervision.

Psychiatric nurse—a registered nurse (RN) who specializes in treating children and adults with emotional or behavior disorders.

Therapist—can refer to any of the above professionals, if they do psychotherapy.

Psychopharmacologist—an MD experienced in the use of psychiatric medications. Unfortunately, many MDs are not fully skilled in this area.

Over the last thirty years, many doctors have bemoaned the "deprofessionalization" of medicine, such that *patients* have now become *consumers*, physicians have become healthcare providers, and business models rather than ethical perspectives drive much of healthcare delivery. From my perspective as a doctor, this is not quite as bad as we sometimes make it seem. Yes, business managers and insurance companies often get in the way of high-quality care. But now patients and parents can take a more active part in getting the healthcare they need. This is probably especially important in the areas pertaining to mental healthcare, where, unlike neurosurgery, a given family's values and perspectives have to be taken into account when making healthcare decisions and when working directly with a child, which might mean major changes in family routines. To be aware of and sensitive to these issues is not too much for you to expect from your doctor. Is she up to the task? Most doctors are, or can be, if you give them appropriate support and make your needs and wishes known. You have to start by knowing what you have a right to expect.

What You Should Expect Your Doctor to Do for You

Expert Diagnosis, Sensible Diagnostic Reasoning, and Thoughtful Prognosis

First, your child's doctor can be expected to do a careful, expert assessment of your child and, based on that assessment, provide a diagnosis. She should be able to explain the facts and the reasoning that led to this diagnosis and her certainty of the diagnosis. This should be communicated in sensible, easily understood terms. In addition, she should be able to explain to you her estimate of your child's prognosis, or prediction of how your child might fare over the course of development. Complete certainty of a child's future outcomes is never ironclad, however, so treat any prognostic statements with caution. There is a lot you can do to maximize your child's likelihood of a good outcome. In fact, most children with ADHD turn out reasonably well, and the fact that you are reading this book and going to this extra effort to educate yourself is a sure sign of improved odds for your child.

If the doctor is unduly pessimistic about your child's outcomes, talk with other parents who have "been there, seen it, done it." Said one mother: "The best advice I got from another mom with a child with ADHD was that 'moms know their child better than anyone.' If what a physician was doing to or for your child or for the parents didn't 'feel' right, it probably wasn't. She said that doctors are like teachers in that there are some great ones and some really awful ones." Ultimately, there is always something you can do, and continuing to hold fond hopes for your child's outcomes is an important behavior. Remember, ADHD in and of itself does not define or limit what that child can become. "Don't let other people tell you that your child isn't good enough," attests one parent. "Schools, teachers, extended family, soccer coaches, churches and Sunday school teachers, etc., may all say this at one time or another; don't believe them! Just look for other opportunities where you child can succeed!"

Other Diagnostic Conditions: Comorbidities

You have the right to expect that your child's doctor will share information with you about any other disorders your child may have, so-called morbidities, such as learning disabilities, depression, oppositional defiant disorder, and so on. The doctor will often have information available from his professional society (such as the American Academy of Pediatrics) or other sources. He may be able to refer you to additional information sources, some local and some national, 800 numbers, Web pages, and parent support organizations. Information on the common co-occurring conditions in kids with ADHD is listed in Appendix G, but the information you may receive from the doctor is worth noting, since it will likely reflect his or her approach to treating and managing ADHD.

Accurate Information about Causes of ADHD

Your child's doctor should be up to date about possible causes of ADHD. A lot of research is going on, and by explaining the role of genetic factors and environmental causes, your child's doctor should be able to help you understand that

---

Things You Should Expect from Your Doctor

- Careful, expert assessment and diagnosis
- Explanation of the rationale and thinking behind the diagnosis
- Information about your child's future possibilities ("prognosis") and "comorbidities"
- Current thinking about causes
- Information about medication benefits and risks
- Information about behavior therapy
- Tools and toolkits
- Careful monitoring and follow-up
- Referrals and access to other professionals
- Letters of support for needed school services
- Respect for your role as a key member of your child's treatment team
- Willingness to co-construct a treatment plan with you

you're not to blame. She should also be able to warn you off the latest faddish explanations for ADHD, thus sparing you expense and time wasted chasing bogus information. If your doctor encourages you to investigate some such cause, and wants to bill you for the process, get a second opinion, read up on the topic from respected scientific sources (see Chapter 4), and get a new doctor if in fact the whole things turns out to be unfounded. Likewise, your doctor should be the last one to encourage you to spend money, usually not reimbursed by your insurance company, on fancy lab tests, brain scans, or computer programs. Solid scientific studies have yet to establish any value for such procedures, other than for research. At this point in our knowledge, anyone who says otherwise is selling something.

Thorough Explanation of the Proposed Treatment and Diligent Follow-Up

Medication Information

Often the information provided by the doctor will include materials about the role of medications in treating ADHD. Remember that such information is sometimes provided by for-profit companies who want to sell you or your doctor something, usually, but not always, medication of one type or another. This information is usually of high quality and may be reviewed by the Food and Drug Administration (FDA) to ensure that it is not misleading. Nonetheless, such materials will be more likely to emphasize what their sponsor is trying to sell you or your child's doctor.

So read carefully and pay attention to who sponsors the information, whether it be a drug company, a maker of special equipment, or a publisher of testing materials. Information about medication that you receive from your child's doctor will usually include facts about risks and side effects, and how you can know what they are, how to manage such side effects, and information on the risks and benefits of medication, long-term effects, and so on. Realize, of course, that any information you receive from the doctor is just a useful starting point; you will also want to gather additional information that your child's doctor may not have. See the "Taking Charge" section that follows for suggestions.

Behavior Therapy

Your child's doctor should also be able to provide some information about the use and usefulness of behavioral therapies in managing ADHD, and what you need to do to implement such treatments. This form of therapy requires a lot of special effort on your part, however, and very often the regular primary care provider may not have sufficient information and materials available on this treatment. Specialists, such as behavioral pediatricians or child psychiatrists, will often have more information available, but any single source of information is likely not to have all of the kinds of tools that you will eventually want to use. For example, school psychologists, teachers, counselors, special education teachers, and even your minister or rabbi may also have useful information, as well as resources to offer you, in terms of behavioral therapy. This is important, since children needing behavior therapy

> ### Getting the Facts
> ### about Your Child's Treatment
>
> - **Take notes.** Writing down what your provider says will help you remember what you need to know about your child's treatment.
> - **Make a list of questions ahead of time.** Asking your provider questions may be difficult at first. Writing down your questions before you meet with your provider will make asking the questions easier.
> - **Repeat what you hear.** If you're having a complicated discussion with your provider, it may be helpful to repeat what you hear in your own words. This is a good way of confirming that you understood what the doctor said.
> - **Keep a file.** Keep all the important documents related to your child's treatment in an easy-to-access file or binder. Review this binder periodically to make sure you have all the important facts related to your child's treatment.

can have this treatment delivered in different settings: home, school, playground, day camp, and so on. If your child's problems are greatest in the school setting, the ideal persons to provide and implement the behavior therapy will be one of the above school personnel listed earlier. But if your child's behavioral problems are most severe at home, it is likely that you and a private psychotherapist will be doing most of the work. The point here is, you will have to do some of your own research to find the kinds of information and resources that will work best for you.

A few other pointers: remember that behavior therapy is not very effective for inattentive symptoms per se. Such problems are usually better addressed by medication. But behavior therapy can be quite effective for a child's overt behavior problems, such as getting out of one's seat, failing to take turns, fighting, sibling rivalry, or refusing to obey adults' requests. So, depending on the type of problem your child has (e.g., home vs. school), you may need to direct your attention to obtaining a form of behavioral therapy specific to that setting. Several books on behavioral therapy listed in Appendix E provide additional information on who, where, when, and how one best does behavioral therapy.

Tools and Toolkits

Also, you can expect that your child's doctor or therapist will have "tools" or toolkits available to assist in managing your child's ADHD. Such tools and kits might include behavior problem and ADHD *symptom checklists* that can be used by you or your child's teachers to track the type and severity of symptoms your child may experience. He may also have informational videotapes, sample charts to monitor and reward your child's appropriate behavior, stickers or other small rewards for your child, information sheets for you or your child's teacher, tips about managing ADHD, or even information concerning your child's educational rights.

You will want to keep all of these materials organized, initially placing them in your file cabinet in a place where you can find them. Try not to simply throw all information into a single folder in the file cabinet; it will be hard to remember who gave you that information later. So before filing it, review the information for its helpfulness to you and your family. Write a note on a yellow sticky pad, noting (1) when it was received, (2) who gave it to you, and (3) any points you want to remember about its value to you and your family. If you can't find any value in it, either throw it away *now* (you will have more than enough of such information, and collecting too much of it will often prove overwhelming later) or put it in a special folder entitled "Uncertain value," where you can review it at your leisure (huh?) later on an intermittent basis.

Monitoring and Follow-Up

You can and should expect your doctor to provide what research has shown to be an essential component of long-term quality care: *regular visits, careful monitoring, and follow-up*. Research that colleagues and I have been involved with has shown that regular visits to track your child's progress are keys to quality care. Unfortunately, in many situations, children with ADHD are seen only once or twice a year. This is insufficient, just as such low-level monitoring of juvenile diabetes would be inappropriate. When a child is first diagnosed and treatment has been started, the doctor's seeing the child every two to three weeks is optimal, not just to address any concerns you may have, but also to monitor side effects when medication is used, to obtain feedback and follow-up information from your child's teacher(s), and to ensure that the child's response to treatment has been optimal. Ideally, your child's medication should be adjusted so that he experiences virtually no ADHD symptoms. Sometimes parents are concerned about medication, using as little as possible, but research has shown that "undertreatment" with ADHD medications (using them at doses too low or only sporadically) results in worse longer term outcomes in home, school, and peer-relationship settings.

Careful medication monitoring also means fairly frequent visits, so the doctor can reevaluate your child's response based on feedback from you and your child's teachers, and also by visiting with your child. She can then adjust the medication if necessary and discuss with you any other possible modifications of the treatment approach. Eventually, as your child is doing well, less frequent visits are possible but still should occur at least every three months. Remember, children with ADHD are at risk for developing a range of other conditions, so you'll need careful monitoring and ongoing management throughout your child's adolescence to ensure optimal outcomes in most cases.

Referrals to Specialists

"There is no one doctor that seems to understand all the complexities of ADHD," bemoaned one parent. "I wish someone had told us that ADHD is seldom the sole issue you're going to have to deal with." When more difficult problems arise, such as school failure, depression, or conduct problems, your child's doctor should be able to make a referral to a specialist such as a child psychiatrist or psychologist, or another type of therapist (see Glossary of Practitioner Types, pp. 87–88). Don't be afraid of this, or of asking for such a referral. Sometimes a well-intentioned primary care provider may delay such a referral, perhaps not wanting to offend you. But don't hesitate to press your case if your instincts tell you otherwise, or that the primary care doctor's efforts are not enough to ensure an optimal outcome for your child. His referral is of value nonetheless, since he may have a good working relationship with a specialist in your area, and you may want to capitalize on this.

Other referrals can be necessary as well, such as to a *speech and language therapist* (many children with ADHD have speech and language problems). Referrals to psychologists for purposes of doing intensive psychological and educational testing are also common and are often necessary to determine fully the level of your child's educational needs or to make the case with the school when additional school resources are needed, yet the school is dragging its feet. And, of course, referrals for some type of psychotherapy may occur. There is a large array of different types of specialists who provide some form of therapy. *Caveat emptor*, "let the buyer beware," applies here, since there are vast differences in what passes for therapy from practitioner to practitioner, even among practitioners with the same type of degree and initials after their name. "We visited six therapists before finding one we thought could help us at all," attests one mother. "I find there are not many good therapists around, or doctors either," agreed another.

> "I have been driving my son's treatment, suggesting things, etc. I found someone who could diagnose him to get the ball rolling, but it's been piecemeal finding programs/doctors since then. I never felt blamed by any professional I spoke with, but I did sense their unease over my presenting them with ADHD symptoms. I went to a local mental health clinic to deal with my child's anxiety and worry, and they refused to acknowledge his ADHD as a primary symptom. I now realize they had no expertise in the area."

From another parent:

> "I have found the one single word that has been *key* to all my solutions was *psychopharmacology*. It is medication treatment without psychiatric babble. The only such office located in my insurance plan (for children age twelve and older) happened to be the one that gave me the most effective medication care in a matter of six weeks. They truly know their meds. As someone who totally lost all faith in all insurance companies and my whole state, to say that I am going to take my daughter from a well-known hospital in another state to this psychopharmacologist's office in my own state close by, proves that the system can, and does work—but it works better if you are over twelve years old."

Other types of help, not just for your child, may also be necessary: "Seek family counseling from a good child therapist/psychologist as needed to be able to voice

---

What You Should Expect from a Therapist for Your Child

- Answers to your questions pertaining to his or her credentials, training in behavioral therapy, and experience in treating ADHD children
- Candid discussion of what appears to be "the problem," as well as the goals and methods of therapy
- Direct answers to your questions, as long as they don't compromise some important aspect of the child's confidence
- Candid discussion of the likely length of the treatment
- Use of scientifically proven behavioral treatments for your child's ADHD symptoms
- A positive and understanding relationship with you and your child
- Being treated as a partner in the treatment program
- Absence of blame
- Protection of you and your family's privacy
- Copies of his or her treatment summaries and reports

---

your frustrations and learn to deal with your child's behavior," advises one parent. So what can and should you expect from a therapist? See the accompanying box for some of the highlights. If you find you or your child doesn't establish a positive relationship with the therapist within the first three or four sessions, you may need to seek another one. Older notions of the need to discuss your childhood, your relationships with your own parents, and so forth, are somewhat outdated, so look out if you find that this becomes the major focus of your work together.

Help with Your Administrative Needs

Records and Reports

You can and should expect your doctor and your child's therapist to provide you a written report for your own records. In today's mobile society, documentation of tests and evaluations is essential, can save you the expense of repeating earlier tests, and can enhance the quality of future care, so later healthcare providers will be able to determine exactly what has and has not been done previously.

Letters of Support or Other Communications

Your child's pediatrician and therapist should be prepared to supply various letters of support and other documentation of your child's problems upon request. If your child has to see the school nurse to receive medication during the school day, the doctor will need to confirm that in a letter or form, as required by many school districts. (Increasingly, however, this may not be necessary, now that effective once-a-day medications have become available.) You may also need proof of your child's

ADHD diagnosis for school personnel to conduct the necessary meetings to determine your child's eligibility for additional educational resources. In addition, the doctor's and therapist's documentation of your child's level of difficulties or disabilities will usually be very helpful in obtaining additional school supports. For example, if your child has speech and language problems, and the physician's letter notes the need for twice-weekly speech therapy, you have a very powerful piece of medical evidence working on your behalf. Or if the physician's letter recommends a special education evaluation or specialized classroom placement, you already have a leg up in obtaining these types of additional school resources for your child. Sometimes a physician or therapist will even join a school staffing meeting, either in person (rare) or by conference call (I do this often, when needed). Again, the physician's and/or therapist's presence, whether by letter, by phone, or in person, can really get the system to attend carefully to your child's needs.

Respect for Your Role, Willingness to Form a Partnership

You can and should expect the doctor to *treat you and your opinion with respect.* He should clearly convey his belief that your role is essential, even central, to the overall success of your child's management plan. Here's a good example of this attitude in action from one parent: "The best thing our doctor told us was that if we needed help, we should ask for it—because there was always something we could figure out together that could help. The worst thing we could do would be to allow ourselves to become so frustrated with his behaviors that we would stop loving our child." Without this collaboration, you are likely to feel unsupported and uncertain about what is needed for your child's optimal long-term management.

If your doctor doesn't fit this bill, you're not alone. From time to time parents may have to shop around to find a doctor that really works for their family:

> "The first therapists (at age four) we saw were discouraging about medication and believed that I needed better parenting skills. The first psychiatrist (at age seven) put our daughter on the wrong med. The doctors at the hospital were very good at diagnosing her condition and putting her on the right combination of meds. Another therapist (we saw her only once) told us point blank that she didn't believe in the bipolar diagnosis and kept implying that my child was sexually abused. The next psychiatrist was OK, though he didn't seem very knowledgeable about treating a bipolar/ADHD child."

Even when a doctor is perfectly competent and knowledgeable, if you and the doctor can't form a reasonable partnership, all that competence may go to waste, because it will be hard for you to use. "The child has to connect with the therapist; otherwise it doesn't work," says one parent. "The doctor must take the time to find out what specific problems your child with ADHD is having, as each child has challenges in different areas. The challenges are not all the same and change with the age of the child as well." Which leads us to the next point—finding the right doctor.

Finding the Right Doctor

I can't tell you how often I've heard stories like this: "That doctor told me that I was too overprotective. He also told us that we should just let our son fail. He made me feel like the worst parent in the world." If you've been on the receiving end of this kind of treatment, rest assured that there are plenty of tales like these, too:

> "Our best doctor, before giving us the diagnosis, said, 'Congratulations! You have a healthy child! He doesn't have a brain tumor, he doesn't have cancer, and his vital organs are all OK! He runs and he talks a blue streak. He should live to be a very old man. It is important that you remember this! He does have a condition, however. He has ADD, attention deficit disorder. He will be a lot more challenging than other kids, but he is healthy! Be thankful. You have a great kid.' After twenty years, I can still remember that."

> "Our best doctor gave us the best advice. . . . He encouraged us to get respite help and not to lose sight of our marriage. He explained why it was so important that parents work as a team with kids like Joey. He always talked with Joey during appointments and asked about his perceptions of how things were going. He always told us what a great kid he could be—and that we needed to keep him involved in things and find the things that he was good at . . . that we should never let Joey fail, and we should not lose faith in him."

> "Our doctor explained why it was so important that parents work as a team with kids like Mark. He always talked with Mark on appointments and asked him how things were going. He always told us what a great kid he could be—and that we needed to keep him involved in things and find the things that he was good at."

Finding one of these gems may not be easy, as you may already have found out. "It took at least ten or more times before we found the right combination of physicians that work with us," related one mother. "We have changed doctors a couple of times," said another. "We have paid out of pocket when the HMO doctors were not knowledgeable about ADHD. We have also changed social workers for counseling. You have to get a good fit with your child for them to respond."

Here are some tips for finding the best doctors available.

Checking Your Doctor's Credentials and Training

There is an old medical school joke that goes like this: "What do you call the medical student who graduates from the bottom of his or her medical school class?" The answer: "Doctor!" The point is one you probably already know through experience: Not all doctors are created equal. Like any group of professionals, each doctor comes with his own special strengths and weaknesses, areas where he is especially well trained and areas where he is not. If at all possible, you will need to get a good handle on the strengths and weaknesses of the doctors you choose for your child.

Questions to Ask Your Doctor or His Staff

- Where did you go to medical school? When did you graduate? Where was your internship? In what states do you hold or have you held a license?
- Did you complete a residency? In what specialty area? Are you "board certified"?
- How much experience do you have in diagnosing and treating ADHD? And how many children have you treated?
- Have you taken any other trainings or certifications in diagnosing and treating ADHD?
- What treatments do you provide? Do you provide both behavioral and medication treatments?
- If you don't do both, do you have close colleagues that you work with who can provide the other forms of treatment?

It may be difficult to ask these questions over the phone, but as a minimum, you should be sure to ask them on the first visit, or even ask the receptionist prior to the visit. Some states (like New York, where I live) even allow you to look up the doctor's name on the Web, ascertaining some basic facts about his or her date and place of graduation from medical school, board certifications, and the like. Use Google (*www.google.com*), entering in the name of the state, doctor, and licensing, and see what you can come up with. In addition, some organizations, like the American Academy of Child and Adolescent Psychiatry (*www.aacap.org*) allow you to look up doctors in your geographic area and determine their areas of practice and special interest. In most states, as well as through the American Medical Association (*www.ama.org*), you can also determine whether your state's physician licensing board has taken any disciplinary actions against a physician you are considering.

The lowest level of training that one can complete and still be eligible to practice medicine is to (1) graduate from medical school; (2) complete a one-year internship (usually working in a hospital under supervision, while gaining additional experience); (3) take special examinations recognized by the state in which one wants to practice medicine; and (4) then become a general practitioner licensed to practice general medicine in that particular state only. At the second level, the doctor also completes a residency in a given specialty area, and at the highest level, the doctor takes the test hosted by other doctors from that specialty area, called a "Specialty Board," sponsored by an independent body such as the American Board of Pediatrics, the American Board of Psychiatry and Neurology, the American Board of Family Medicine, and so forth. These special examinations are quite competitive, and only about half of the physicians in any given specialty will have taken and passed their specialty boards.

If you can get a doctor who has completed this level of training and certification, you are off to a good start, but it doesn't guarantee the expertise you need for your child. A pediatrician who is board certified may still have little experience in treating ADHD. Some residencies may provide relatively little training in the areas in which your child needs special competence. Many times, a doctor can take continuing medical education courses and seminars, and get the necessary additional experience she needs. Other times, a physician may simply acquire lots of experience, just by reading lots of journals, keeping up with new research, and treating lots of kids. Likewise, a physician might be "only" a general practitioner but still have all the necessary skills to do a very competent job in diagnosing and treating a child with ADHD. But you should look for all of these clues of competence and ask whatever questions you need to assure yourself that your doctor has all of the tools and knowledge at her disposal to work on behalf of your child and family. In some instances, you may want to go with a particular doctor even though she may not have been fully trained in a given area of practice, particularly if she has been recommended by multiple parents who are satisfied customers.

Sources of Referrals to Good Doctors

In my experience, the single best source of names of doctors that will fill your needs is other parents—those who have been in your position, who differ only in that they are a few years further along than you. Parent groups such as CHADD (*www.chadd.org*), NAMI (*www.nami.org*), and Federation for Families (*www.ffcmh.org*), all of which have state and local chapters, will be your single best source of names. Likewise, family friends, particularly those who have had a child with similar difficulties, are an excellent resource. Or if you are looking for a specialist, such as a child psychiatrist, behavioral pediatrician, or psychologist, you may find that your primary care doctor can provide some good names, with the added advantage that she has professional relationships with these persons.

Another approach is to use one of the online services that lets you identify doctors in your area, based on specialty, age, gender, time since medical school, place of training, board certification, history of any disciplinary actions or complaints, and so forth. For only $10 you can get a list of up to twenty doctors by going to the website *www.healthgrades.com*. And last, a number of websites of parent and professional associations will give names of professionals in your area. This "sight-unseen approach" is the least preferable option and should be used only when you have exhausted all other options. As one mother pointed out, sometimes doctors you find on websites don't list ADHD as their specialty but, more often, might note only that they deal with "mental health issues." One further approach is to seek out a university with specialty expertise in ADHD, such as found in the CHADD National Resource Center of ADHD (*www.help4adhd.org/en/treatment/prof*).

Cultivating a Good Parent–Professional Partnership

Even once you've found a qualified doctor with experience in ADHD (and any other problems your child has), you need to find out whether you two can form an effective partnership on behalf of your child. Just as in any relationship, developing trust and teamwork takes time. So it may not be clear right off whether you can form a partnership. But you can start to get a sense of whether this partnership will work. Does your child's doctor seem put out or irritated when you ask about his background and training? If so, this is not a good start. Does your child's doctor seem defensive or irritated when you share information you have found in your readings or on the Web? Is she patient and happy to answer questions you may have? Does she ask about your concerns and questions about her diagnosis and assessment, or try to find out if you have any worries about treatments that she has recommended? If so, these are good signs. She is obviously trying to make sure that what she is doing is going to be in sync with you, your understanding of your child's needs, and your overall family issues and challenges.

Links for Finding a Doctor

- American Academy of Child and Adolescent Psychiatry: *www.aacap.org*
- American Psychiatric Association: *www.psych.org/apa_members/db_info.cfm*
- American Academy of Pediatrics: *www.aap.org/referral*
- American Academy of Neurology: *www.aan.com/public/find.cfm*
- American Medical Association: *www.ama-assn.org/aps/amahg.htm*
- National Association of Social Workers: *www.socialworkers.org*
- CHADD: *www.chadd.org*
- Child and Adolescent Bipolar Foundation: *www.bpkids.org*
- American Psychological Association: *helping.apa.org/find.html*

As a general rule, doctors, like anyone else, want to do a good job and to be appreciated for it. Not all doctors will have much experience in such partnerships, however, and you may have to "break them in." So remember, a partnership is a two-way street, and this means you have to listen to the doctor and try to understand what he tells you, just as you want the same from him. Here are a few basic principles for forming effective parent–provider partnerships.

Participate!

An effective parent–provider partnership demands active participation from both parents and providers:

- *Speak up.* Let your child's providers know that you want to take an active role in your child's treatment. At first, you may find this difficult, but with practice and support you can learn to approach your child's providers with ease. But don't just make this sound demanding; ask what role the doctor would like you to play. If he makes it sound minimal, you have an opening to say you're willing and eager to do more.
- *Provide information.* You know a lot about your child, but sometimes you do not have the opportunity to share your knowledge with your child's provider. You should be sure to tell your child's provider all that you can about your child's history, symptoms, needs, and so forth.

Know Your Rights

Most public mental health agencies list your rights as a consumer of health and mental health services in a document entitled the Patient's Bill of Rights. You should obtain this document, review it, and take appropriate action if you feel the rights of your child are being violated. If an agency or private provider doesn't have a Patient's Bill of Rights, ask them to make one. In addition, check out the Patient's Bill of Rights at *www.psych.org/public_info/men_insurance.cfm*, a joint initiative of all major mental health professional organizations.

Get the Facts

You must get accurate information about your child's condition and treatment. This requires asking a lot of questions. If you don't understand something a provider has said, ask questions until it becomes clear. Doctors and other healthcare providers will assume a parent understands unless he or she lets the provider know otherwise.

Remember That Parents Are Experts Too

As a parent, you are the most knowledgeable expert concerning your child, his development, strengths, assets, and special challenges. You have much more opportunity to know and observe your child than a provider does and can provide valuable information about your child's functioning. Of course, you must also get input and advice from others, but if you are told something that does not fit with your prior experiences, ask questions and explain to the doctor or healthcare professional why you feel as you do.

Know Your Limits

In addition to realizing that you, too, are an expert in your child's treatment, you must know your limits when it comes to collaborating with your child's provider. You must negotiate and openly discuss your role in your child's treatment with the provider, but you should be careful not to assume more responsibilities than you are capable of performing. Trying to do everything right, it is all too easy to get overwhelmed, as one mother described:

"I was using many tools and behavior modification techniques I'd learned about at CHADD, but things were not working at all. I was extremely resistant to the idea of using medication, because I knew that Ritalin was a stimulant, plus I had a sister-in-law who (I know now) overdosed her hyperactive son until he was a zombie. However, I was at the end of my rope. Jonathan was losing interest in school, and he had been an excellent and eager student in early elementary. I scheduled an appointment with his pediatrician and went in with a folder full of documentation. Based on my input and documentation from teachers, she suggested we do a trial of Ritalin that very day. Having exhausted all other avenues, I hesitantly sent him off to school the next day with a ten-milligram dose after breakfast. After school that afternoon, Jonathan was able to tell me for the first time what went on in school that day. His first statement, though, had me nearly in tears: 'Mom, we had a spelling test today, and the teacher asked us to look over our papers before handing them in. When I looked at my paper, I remembered writing the words! I've never done that before.' I now compare my denying Jonathan Ritalin up to this time to denying eyeglasses to one who is nearsighted, all the while commanding that if he would only try harder to see, he could."

Recognize Efforts by Professionals

Show your appreciation to your child's healthcare providers. Providers enjoy receiving positive feedback. Such feedback can help establish and maintain a healthy respect and working relationship. After you have finished working with a provider, consider keeping in touch. Due to the usually time-limited involvement providers have with families, they often have no knowledge as to how events have unfolded and are genuinely interested in hearing from former patients and families. Or even, how about just saying to the doctor, "You've been so terrific and we're really grateful. Is there anything I can do for you?" Another parent noted:

> "We parents sometimes forget that we can offer 'professional' courtesies in return. I am an editor and once had a doctor who needed an editor, so I offered to refer him to someone who could help him with papers. . . . I found this was a good way to offer a gesture of appreciation *and* a way to put the doctor on notice that I considered myself his equal, willing and able to reciprocate. I think this can go a long way toward dispelling any vestige of paternalism."

Communicate Clearly and Assertively

Don't go from the frying pan to the fire. Doctors are people, too, and you don't want to find yourself in a situation where you have alienated the only doctor in town . . . unless you're ready to move! If you basically respect your doctor's expertise, or if she is willing to learn more about what is needed to give your child the best care, you may have the makings of a good partnership over time. But you have to state your needs and wishes clearly and nonargumentatively to win the doctor over to your team.

EXERCISE 1

Practice these phrases at home before trying them out on your doctor:

- How we can we be certain that my son's problem is not just a learning disability?

    Or

- How can we know the difference between this and oppositional defiant disorder, which I have heard so much about?

Or

- Can you say more about why you considered this diagnosis but not
_____?

    Or

- I appreciate the workup you've done, but I still have some worries about the diagnosis, and it seems to me that there may be other things going on. Is there any additional evaluation we can do?

    Or

- Do you have a colleague you can refer me to who might be willing to take a second look?

Avoid blaming the doctor or using sentences that begin with "You should . . ." or "You ought to . . ." or "You aren't doing . . ." Communicate clearly but in a nonhostile fashion, more along the line of "I was hoping you might be willing . . ." or "What do you think about . . . ?" or "I wonder if we did . . ." or "Would you mind if I . . . ?" If you had to be particularly assertive on one visit and wonder if you touched a nerve in the doctor, but you think there are still basic ingredients of his wanting to do right by you and your child, send a follow-up note, perhaps with a plate of cookies or box of doughnuts. Again, doctors are people, too. I am one, and I am quite sure of it.

To give you a firmer sense of the ground on which you are standing, it might be helpful to check out several organizations' professional standards for the diagnosis and treatment of ADHD at the National Resource Center on ADHD, supported by the Centers for Disease Control (CDC) and hosted by CHADD, *www.help4adhd.org/en/treatment/guides*. Be sure of what you need and communicate it clearly. In the event that you feel the doctor has breached some major professional standard, and you have not achieved any satisfactory resolution to the problem and are concerned that others might encounter the same problems and possible dangers, you may need to consider filing a complaint. First discuss it with another savvy parent, and if it still makes sense, you can make contact with all states' professional licensing boards online at *www.noah-health.org/english/usdoctors.html*, a free service provided by the New York Online Access to Health. This site is also chock-full of other useful information and various state and national website links.

Taking Charge: How to Get What You Need from the Doctor

Knowing what you have a right to expect from your child's doctor may give you the confidence to go after it when it's not forthcoming. But how do you give yourself the best possible chance of getting results? The following pages offer tips and ideas—from parents, as well as professionals—for actions to take and resources to tap when you have problems with the diagnosis delivered by the doctor or the treatment recommended.

Resolving Problems with the Diagnosis and Prognosis

Are you worried that the diagnosis the doctor has made is inaccurate or incomplete, or that the diagnostic process wasn't thorough enough? Unclear on the reasoning that led to the diagnosis? Dissatisfied with the doctor's explanation of the course of ADHD or uncomfortable with the prognosis? First, remember the principle of clear and assertive communication. Explicitly state your questions to the doctor: "Doctor, can you tell me more about the diagnostic process itself? I am unclear about how much certainty we can have about the diagnosis given that so much is simply based on observation and teacher's ratings, and the like. How can we be sure? Can you tell me more about your rationale for this diagnosis, rather than [some other diagnosis or concern you have]?"

For most of us, these phrases or questions will not come naturally, since it might seem like we're second-guessing the doctor. So for starters, write the phrase or question down, perhaps beginning with "I am concerned about . . ." or "I was wondering . . ." Then state your question more explicitly, such as in the earlier examples in Exercise 1, where the question tends to be open-ended: "Can you say more about . . . ?" or "How can we be sure . . . ?" Once it is well stated, in a way that your candid but friendly critics don't think is hostile, practice saying it—in front of a mirror, with your spouse, or with a best friend. Anticipate a vague or noncommittal response from the doctor and then develop a follow-up, such as "I understand better now; thanks for explaining. But I still feel like we need to look further into this. What else might you recommend?" If the doctor is still noncommittal or vague, repeat the phrase, using the "broken record technique": "I understand what you're saying, but I still wonder if. . . . What can we do to further explore . . . ?" Or more daring still: "I agree that there probably isn't a learning disability, but from what I have been reading, psychological testing is sometimes needed to firmly rule out that possibility. Would you be willing to write a letter to the school requesting that they do this?"

Most doctors will figure out that you're serious, and if you remain pleasant throughout, you can usually get some good degree of cooperation, additional explanation, or other assistance. But what if that doesn't work? Here, you may have to do some additional homework:

• Do additional study about the question you have (See Chapter 4 and Appendices E and I for leads to good sources).

• Know the state of the art for diagnosing ADHD, so you don't make unrealistic demands on the doctor. Studies are actively under way to determine whether the diagnostic process can be made more accurate through the use of computerized performance tests, brain scans, blood tests, or even genetic screens, but we are not there yet. In addition, researchers are attempting to determine the best ways to help doctors become more reliable in their approach, so that they will be less prone either to under- or overdiagnosis. For example, a Presidential Commission recently recommended schoolwide screening for all children and youth, to reduce the number of children who are missed, not only those with ADHD, but also children with other conditions, such as depression.

• Talk to other parents who are experienced in the area with their own children. If you don't know any, you can usually find some by locating the closest parent support group near you at *www.chadd.org*, *www.ffcmh.org*, or *www.nami.org*, or by contacting your state's parent training and information centers and community parent resource centers, with each state's contact information found at *www.taalliance. org/PTIs.htm.*

• Check standards for assessment from practice guidelines, as described earlier (see *www.help4adhd.org/en/treatment/guides*).

• Ask explicitly for additional tests that you feel might be warranted. If the doctor declines, ask for his rationale.

• Read in the *Diagnostic and Statistical Manual of Mental Disorders* (fourth edition, text revision [DSM-IV-TR] American Psychiatric Association, American Psychiatric Press, Inc., Washington, DC, 2000). Most public libraries will have this available, and most of DSM-IV-TR can be found online, simply by typing "DSM-IV" and the specific diagnosis name into *www.google.com*. Quite reader-friendly and downloadable versions of the DSM criteria can be found at *www.nimh.nih.gov/publicat/index.cfm* or *www.healthplace.com*, while the exact criteria wording can be found on the Internet Mental Health site at *www.mentalhealth.com*.

• Go back and ask the doctor again!

• Ask for a copy of the child's medical record.

• Review the principles of action (see Chapter 2). Do you need to change course or map out a new strategy?

• Go to one of the online chat rooms, starting first with *www.chadd.org* (CHADD Chat), *www.nami.org* (NAMI's Online Communities), or those available through MSN or AOL, or *www.healthyplace.com*.

• And when all else has failed get a second opinion and consider seeking another doctor (see earlier links for finding a doctor).

Reconciling Conflicts or Gaps in Information

If you're actively gathering information during the diagnostic (and then treatment) process, at some point you're going to run into something that conflicts with what your doctor has told you or that he hasn't mentioned at all. How do you reconcile the information the doctor has given you with what you've heard elsewhere?

• First, and foremost, talk to the doctor. Be respectful but assertive. If you find some useful information pertaining to the discrepancy, particularly if it is information prepared by that doctor's own association (*www.aap.org*, *www.aacap.org*, or *www.apa.org*), bring that printed material to his attention. One parent described handling this situation under ideal conditions: "I have been very fortunate in this area and have had access to wonderful and knowledgeable treatment professionals over the years. We have always been a *part* of the team, including my son. When a professional, such as a primary care provider, felt the case was beyond their expertise, they were comfortable saying so. If they didn't seem capable I would have changed. Being educated in the topic, I would have known!"

• To become like the parent just quoted, you may need to do further research. See Appendix E for specific books; also, see the websites listed earlier that may help you reconcile the different pieces of information you have heard. I have given you a fair number of Web-based resources, which can be confusing, but all things being equal, first start with CHADD's home page (*www.chadd.org*), since this organization is focused specifically on ADHD, or turn to its National Resource Center on ADHD (*www.help4adhd.org*) Also check out NIMH information (*www.nimh.nih.gov/publicat/index.cfm*), my own center's (Center for the Advancement of Children's Mental Health) website (*www.kidsmentalhealth.org*), the Facts for Families of the American Academy of Child and Adolescent Psychiatry (*www.aacap.org/publications/factsfam/index.htm*), or scan the latest published research on this topic on PubMed (*www.ncbi.nlm.nih.gov*), as described in Chapter 4.

• This is a good issue to raise with other parents. Find out what they know about it through your local parent group. There is a lot of shared wisdom out there!

• Share an article with the doctor that provides the latest information about the area where he doesn't seem to be knowledgeable (such as the benefits of treating older youth and adults). You might even find an article from the journal of his specialty society, such as the *Journal of Pediatrics*, the *Journal of the American Academy of Child and Adolescent Psychiatry*, or the journal simply called *Pediatrics*. If you're afraid the doctor might think you're trying to show him up, try giving him the article and telling him you don't really understand it but saw it referred to on a parent support website, and wonder if he could help you figure out whether it's pertinent for your son.

• Review the basic principles outlined in Chapter 2. Do you need to map out a new plan of action, such as getting a second opinion, changing doctors, or changing your mind about what you previously thought was the best approach? Have you gone down an incorrect path based on incomplete or discrepant information that you now understand more fully?

• When all else has failed, post your question on a parent website or CHADD's chat room (*www.chadd.org*). Remember, other parents may be your greatest source of help when it seems like nothing else has worked.

It can be difficult to ask doctors what they think about information you've obtained outside their office, without putting them on the defensive. They may read into your queries an implication that they should have been more up to date and/or more forthcoming with you. If you find yourself tongue-tied in these situations, try Exercise 2.

EXERCISE 2

Practice these phrases at home before trying them out on your doctor:

• Doctor, I heard on television about this new diagnostic test for ADHD. What can you tell me about it? Where would you suggest I go to get more information?

    Or

• Doctor, I'm concerned about how well Thomas's diagnosis seems to fit his current problems. I was reading an interesting article on bipolar disorder the

other day and wondered whether this might fit his situation. Can I leave this article with you, and then come back or call you in a few days so we can talk
about it some more? I know you have a lot to worry about, but this will help
me set my mind at ease. Thanks so much.

   Or

- Doctor, Ellen's teacher raised questions about whether she might in fact have a
  learning disability in addition to her ADHD problems. Also, I was reading up
  on tics and ADHD, and wondered if Ellen's constant clicking her tongue might
  be a tic? What do you think? How should we go about having that evaluated?

Sometimes, of course, the doctor simply feels too pressed for time to discuss issues she hadn't planned on getting into at this appointment. So what do you do
when you have some pressing questions that have not yet been answered to your satisfaction? Try Exercise 3, below.

EXERCISE 3

How to Get Your Doctor to Remove His Hand from the Doorknob and Listen When He's Rushing Out

- Doctor, I know you're busy, but can I get you to take a few more minutes before you move on? I have two short questions, and I really need your input on
  them.

   Or

- Doctor, I can see you need to move on. Would it be better for me to talk with
  you later today? Can I call you this afternoon at a specific time, or can you call
  me? Or would you prefer to try to tackle these questions now?

Addressing Treatment Concerns: Problems and Potential Solutions

As mentioned under "Things You Should Expect from Your Doctor," you should be
prepared to gather information about medications (and other therapies) that your
doctor doesn't have or doesn't offer. Again, you'll find this information in the
sources listed in Appendices E and I and on the various websites I've given you.

The Medication Decision

Whether to allow your child to be treated with medication for ADHD is always a
tough decision. You can make it with confidence by following the advice in this book
on getting the best possible information from your child's doctor and from independ-

ent sources. Here is input from two other sources: parents who have already made the decision, and Harold Koplewicz, the founder/director of the New York University Child Study Center and author of the widely praised book *It's Nobody's Fault: New Hope and Help for Difficult Children and Their Parents*.

Parents Talk about Using Medication for ADHD

"I feel so frustrated and so angry when people (in friendly and social gatherings) say, "Don't put your kid on medication" or, "If only that parent would discipline her kid, that child wouldn't need to be on medication." People who say things like that either don't yet have children of their own, or don't have children with ADHD. Accepting that Roberta needs medication and will probably be on it for years has made the biggest difference in our family."

"The teachers really seem to push the most of anyone for medicine, so they have do not have to deal with any behavior/school problems."

"I do not like the fact that she is tied to four medications a day for her to function."

"I am sick and tired of people who do not know what they are talking about speaking out against the use of ADHD medication. It has been a godsend for my son, and I get really angry when people say what he really needs is good parenting."

"We have been criticized for having our child on medications, most recently by a private pediatrician, but the good news is: She's happy. She loves middle school. She is on the Honor Roll, plays on school sports teams, and seems to be accepted by the kids. She has new friends, but she still longs to have a best friend."

"My daughter has a better teacher this year, more able to adjust to my daughter's hyperactivity. My daughter has also matured and controls her behavior better; therefore, we have been able to take her off medicine, and she is happier/less moody off medicine."

"Studies show that habitual brain functioning with medication increases the actual physical structure of brain connections. Learning this last fact recently at a conference ('Diamonds in the Rough' in Rockville, Maryland) changed my whole view on medication for kids."

"The best advice was trying the medication. That was the hardest step to take: deciding that your six-year-old needs to take a pill every day. I still don't like it."

"The biggest problem is medication management."

(cont.)

Questions to Ask Your Child's Doctor

According to my colleague Harold Koplewicz, it's important to discuss the following questions with your child's provider when any medication is being considered:

- What is the diagnosis?
- What is the medicine, and how does it work?
- Have studies been done on the medication?
- Which tests need to be done before my child starts the medication?
- How soon will I see an improvement?
- How often will my child have to take the medicine?
- How will the decision be made to stop it?
- What are the negative side effects of the medicine?
- What will happen if my child doesn't take it?

But beyond this research, what do you do if your child's doctor or therapist . . .

- *Is not communicating with the school and vice versa?* Acknowledge how busy he is. Consider sharing with him the American Academy of Pediatrics guidelines (*www.help4adhd.org/en/treatment/guides*) about the necessity of getting information and regular communications going between the medical and educational systems. Offer to help by delivering notes or checklists to and from the teacher. If you need the doctor to write up a report or letter to the school to support your request for educational services, it might be helpful under some circumstances if you provide a sample letter, perhaps one obtained from other parents that fits the school district your child is in, or one of the sample letters I have provided in Appendix H. Or if there is a communication problem between the school and the doctor's office, it might help if you work both sides—asking both to call each other or passing on information to each side that the one party is hoping that the other party will call them. Or you might send a letter prior to the visit, saying you are looking forward to getting together and discussing the results of the communication exchange between the two parties you are trying to connect.
- *Does not communicate or collaborate with your child's psychotherapist or doctor?* Speak to both of them, asking each to call the other, making sure they have each other's phone numbers. Repeat the request if needed, and to make it more urgent and immediate, indicate to the doctor that you'll call him the following day to find out "how it went."
- *Hasn't told you enough about his proposal for medication to make you feel comfortable approving this treatment?* See the sidebar on page 89.
- *Hasn't come up with a medication that is effective without intolerable side effects?* This is not necessarily a sign of insufficient knowledge or expertise on the part of the doctor. Often, when one medication does not work or has side effects (this happens

with one-fourth of kids), an excellent response for most of these "nonresponders" can still be achieved with one of the other medications. It's not unusual for several medication trials to be needed before you arrive at the most effective medication, so don't give up or be too concerned about the need for this. If the third medication to be tried has not worked, then it is time to get additional consultation with someone expert in the use of these medications and other various alternatives. See pages 98 and 99 for finding qualified specialists. If the medication is appropriately prescribed and the dose is correct, most children will be able to function with little or no impact due to their ADHD symptoms. *Don't settle for less than this level of response.*

- *Is not up to date on the latest breakthroughs in medications that might potentially help with the child's problems, such as the availability of a new, longer acting medication or one with fewer side effects, and doesn't show any awareness of this possible approach?* Consider sharing the American Academy of Child and Adolescent Psychiatry treatment guidelines for ADHD, available at *www.help4adhd.org/en/treatment/guides*.

- *Seems less concerned than you are about the child's appetite problems or height and weight due to medication?* Download and read CHADD's Fact Sheet No. 3, Medical Management of ADHD (*www.help4adhd.org/en/treatment/medical*), then share and discuss the section on height and weigh with your doctor. Additionally, you can track your child's growth yourself by viewing and downloading the CDC's latest growth charts at *www.cdc.gov/growthcharts*.

- *Hasn't offered much practical help with bothersome medication side effects?* Review the CHADD Fact Sheet No. 3, described earlier. Also consider reading and sharing Tim Wilens's *Straight Talk about Psychiatric Medications for Kids* (New York: Guilford Press, 2004).

- *Hasn't done any blood tests in a while?* Routine blood tests for the stimulant medications are not really necessary, but they can be reassuring (and expensive) for parents. Most other medications might require more

> ### Managing Stimulant Medication Side Effects
>
> - Wait two weeks; sleep and appetite problems often go away.
> - Lower, raise, or change the time of the dose, depending on the side effect.
> - Take medication with food, not on an empty stomach.
> - Consider a change to long-acting medications for side effects on short-acting medications, or vice versa.
> - Add medication to counteract side effects (e.g., clonidine or guanfacine for sleep problems).
> - Change medications if side effects are too bothersome or problematic.

regular blood tests, however. Check on these facts for specific medications at *www.nami.org* or *www.mentalhealth.com*. If blood tests appear warranted, share this information with your doctor, and ask explicitly if blood tests can be done.

- *Always takes the "that's confidential" position with you about your youngster (keeping an older child's confidences), and it's interfering with problem solving and infor-*

mation sharing? It is important for the doctor to keep your youngster's confidence, but she is obligated to inform you if your child is doing something that puts himself or others at serious risk. Acknowledge the doctor's need to keep your child's confidence, but also express your need for her guidance about the best means of working with your child given her additional knowledge about what the child is thinking/feeling. It may help if you set up a private meeting with the doctor, without your youngster, to discuss concerns that you have, then, in that setting, explicitly seek the doctor's advice, based on her best knowledge of the youth.

• *Overemphasizes the disability caused by ADHD, at the expense of the child's self-confidence and self-esteem?* Too often, we doctors forget that if we're always talking about the weaknesses and problems caused by ADHD, the child may begin to think that's all there is to him. "Teach your child that ADHD can be a gift as well as a disability, and point out the many famous people with ADHD who have done great things" was one parent's solution. People who have turned potential disabilities into sources of strength include Roger Bannister, the world's first four-minute miler, who was told he would never walk again after severe burns to the legs; Franklin D. Roosevelt; and Lance Armstrong, who battled and overcame cancer, only to return and repeatedly win the Tour de France, the world's greatest and most strenuous bike race. One parent cited the April 28, 2002, *Fortune* magazine article, "Overcoming Dyslexia," as a reminder of how much kids with disabilities like ADHD can achieve; the article profiles an impressive collection of CEOs and other "movers and shakers" who have struggled throughout life with ADHD and/or learning disabilities. You can really bring your child's potential up close by finding an ADD/ADHD adult who can be a role model for your child, an idea that one parent found invaluable.

• *Gave you simple instructions for using time-out and star charts at home, but now that you've tried it, you find it's much more complicated than you thought and just isn't working?* First, for more comprehensive information on how to put behavior therapy in place for your child, see *Taking Charge of ADHD* by Russell Barkley or *1-2-3 Magic* by Thomas W. Phelan. I've named a number of other texts and offered several useful behavior charts in Appendix I. However, as you have probably figured out, behavior therapy is more complicated than it seems, and it often takes an experienced therapist to "debug" why it seems not to work with a given child. Ask your doctor for a referral to a psychologist who is expert in behavior therapy (many are not, unfortunately). Ask parents in your area who is well qualified in this form of treatment, or use the boxed list, "Links for Finding a Doctor." Also, find and join a parent training group. Many organizations sponsor them, but check first with your local CHADD chapter. That failing, ask your pediatrician, local hospital, church or synagogue. As a final resort, check with the State Resource Directory for Children with Disabilities at *childrenwithdisabilities.ncjrs.org/states.html,* or with your state's Parent Training and Information Centers or Community Parent Resource Centers, accessed though the online directory at *www.taalliance.org/PTIs.htm.*

• *Doesn't think it's his problem when things aren't going well at school?* Again, he's busy. But practice guidelines (*www.help4adhd.org/en/treatment/guides*) are clear about the necessity of teamwork between the doctor and the schools. Offer to help by delivering notes or checklists to and from the teacher, but if the doctor remains resistant, either you are seeing the wrong doctor, or you are going to have to manage this by yourself. Not a good idea.

• *Disagrees with you about medication holidays (summers, weekends)?* In the final analysis, it's your decision. I would recommend that the child remain on medication on weekends and summers if she has significant problems during these time periods, whether it be with sibling relations, parent–child conflict, completing homework, or sitting quietly during religious services. On the other hand, if she gets along with friends and doesn't have particular problems with focus and attention during these periods, stopping the medications during these periods probably is just fine.

• *Doesn't seem to have experience with treating comorbid conditions?* This family's experience is not all that uncommon:

> "My daughter has some undiagnosed mood/personality challenges, and she reacts very adversely to most of the medications that are typically used to treat ADHD. I think these two factors have made it very difficult to find good care. Doctors who have experience treating this type of comorbidity have been very hard to find. I also have felt that several of the doctors I worked with just gave her one med after another, without really trying to understand or address both of her issues. Frankly, I'm still looking for help with her."

For this kind of problem, just as this parent suggested, it's time to get help from someone more expert. Ask your doctor to recommend someone who has had experience in this area. If she gets defensive, this partnership is not going to work very well, so consider a new partner. Finding a new doctor is not easy, as this family describes. Try some of the strategies outlined earlier in this chapter.

• *Strongly recommends a treatment you've never heard of?* Ask the questions listed in "The Medication Decision," page 108 (these can be just as revealing about nonmedication treatments). See the summary of current research-based information on alternative treatments in the sidebar in Chapter 4, page 72.

• *Doesn't want to consider the possibility that the diagnosis is off, even though all the treatments you've tried have failed?* "Our family has a very complex psychiatric medical background," said one mother. "It has been an incredible journey over the past eight years to find a perceptive facility (and/or physician) adept and attentive at sifting through diagnoses to get an accurate view and develop a treatment plan that helps our children live 'normal lives.'" For this problem, a first step might be to try the practice dialogue in Exercise 2 and then to keep trying. Share information on additional disorders that you're concerned about, getting information from *www.nimh.nih.gov/publicat/index.cfm* or my own center's website (*www.kidsmentalhealth.org*).

• *Doesn't seem concerned when you say the medication doesn't seem to be working as well as it did at first?*

1. Don't adjust dosages or stop medication without first consulting your child's healthcare provider.
2. Don't neglect the possibility of using other treatments, such as behavior

therapy, or more fully involving the older child/adolescent as an active participant and decision maker in his or her treatment choices.

3. There are many possible reasons for incomplete or partial response, and you and the child's doctor need to consider them all in determining what to do in response: The medication doses may be too low. Your child is growing and changing, and as her brain matures, different brain chemical systems evolve and "come on line," so a stimulant that didn't work before or caused side effects may now work very well, just like a medication that has worked in the past may no longer work. Or perhaps your child's condition has evolved and what was uncomplicated ADHD is now complicated by mood problems or bipolar disorder. Here are some questions you might ask yourself and your child's doctor if your child's medication no longer seems to be working:

   a. What is your opinion about why the medication doesn't seem to be working anymore?
   b. Do we need to reevaluate the diagnosis? Might it have changed over time?
   c. Do we need to change the dose or increase its frequency?
   d. Is the dose at the maximum level for a child of this age?
   e. What do the research studies suggest one should do for this kind of problem?

• *Doesn't seem to want to change your child's treatment along with his growth and development?* Mickey's mother said, "I've had problems when I wanted to change the strength of the medication. As Mickey grew, I noticed it wasn't doing the job. The doctor has not been real good about wanting to mess with the dosage of the medication." This doctor may need more information about dosing strategies. Share with him the recommendations of the American Academy of Pediatrics concerning treatment and use of medication (*www.help4adhd.org/en/treatment/guides*).

• *Doesn't want to investigate the reasons for worsening of symptoms?* "When our child acted out more seriously several months ago," said one parent, "I attempted to call the doctor; he was out, and when he did call, he just left a message on my phone: 'Increase his medication one tablet.' We and the school didn't think this was the answer." Try some variations on the practice dialogue in Exercise 2, such as "Doctor, I'm concerned that what we've been trying doesn't seem to be working. Could it be that some other problem is going on, perhaps in addition to his ADHD? How can we find out?"

• *Doesn't want to treat an older child with medicine and is unaware of the literature indicating that ADHD is often a lifelong disorder and requires ongoing treatment?* This guy or gal needs additional information. Share the practice guidelines of his or her professional organization (*www.help4adhd.org/en/treatment/guides*) or the informative brochures you can print off of the NIMH website at *www.nimh.nih.gov/publicat/index.cfm*.

• *Is continuing therapy, even though your child doesn't want to see the therapist?* A good therapist is usually flexible and able to respond to a child that is unmotivated or resistant to therapy. Although behavior therapy is the only proven form of therapy for ADHD, children with ADHD often have other problems that may benefit from other treatments, such as individual psychotherapy in one-on-one, private sessions with the child, accompanied by intermittent but general feedback to you. However, if the child does not like the therapist, even after six to eight sessions, it's time to try out another therapist. As one parent put it, "Therapy was fruitless. The child psychologists (I think we tried about seven or eight) could not open the door to Tony, and the adult psychiatrist (once again) was too impressed by Tony's articulate and insightful language. Tony refused to return to him, and since he looked out of the window most of the time that I was in the room, I agreed with Tony."

• *Spends timing talking and playing with your child, but the therapy doesn't seem to be working?* Good therapy depends on good communication and shared understanding of the goals and methods of treatment. That is not always what you get: Many therapists have not been trained in behavior therapy, the only proven form of psychotherapy that works for ADHD and oppositional/aggressive symptoms. Get other parents' advice or seek out someone specifically trained in this area through the Association for the Advancement of Behavior Therapy (*www.aabt.org*).

Getting around Common Roadblocks

Parents talk about certain obstacles over and over. Here are the ones I typically hear that pertain to treatment and how you can surmount them:

• *You've tried everything to deal with really resistant side effects, and now you feel you're left with the choice of living with the side effect or discontinuing the medication and living with the child's untreated symptoms.* Psychiatric medications can be quite complicated, and relatively few physicians are truly expert in using them when snags like this occur. This may involve using several medications in combination or using some medications with which your doctor has no experience. Most likely you will have to consult a child and adolescent psychiatrist who is also expert in ADHD. This may also mean you'll have to travel to a university to get this kind of help. There's a list of such places on the CHADD website (*www.help4adhd.org/en/treatment/prof*).

• *Your child desperately wants to play sports, but his medication effect starts to wear off in the middle of practices, and the timing is such that there's no adult available to administer another dose at the time that would make a difference.* There are now quite a number of longer acting, truly once-a-day medications that can tide a child over these kinds of situations. But if the long-acting medication given in the morning doesn't solve the problem, another strategy might be to use the long-acting medication somewhat later in the day, say, in the late morning or at lunch. This might mean your child will end up taking medication at two times during the day. With these medications, timing is everything (almost).

• *You live in a small town, where there is no one qualified to provide behavior therapy (or the only therapy available has been unsuccessful).* How can you teach yourself to use behavior management techniques without a therapist? For starters, you'll need to read the best books on the subject (see my list in Appendix E). It is also frequently possible to get remote, ongoing help by experienced behavior therapists. For example, you might first need to travel to meet with a competent behavior therapist closest to you (see *www.aabt.org* to find one, or talk with CHADD parents in that city by contacting that city's CHADD group, *www.chadd.org*). Before meeting with the behavior therapist, explain your situation and find out whether she is willing to provide phone therapy (most are). If, after meeting, you find you have hit it off pretty well, set up a regular phone consultation with her. A similar approach might be used with a child psychopharmacologist, who can often set up the medication program and then assist your local provider in managing the medication on an ongoing basis.

• *Your child consistently resists your simplest requests for completing chores at home.* Behavior therapy is designed to address just such problems, yet point systems and other incentives aren't always enough. Parents often need to be more creative, and an understanding of how your child's mind works due to ADHD will serve as the foundation for effective ideas. Here's an example from Seth, the father of seven-year-old Sam:

> "The best advice I ever got was a psychologist explaining to me how his brain processes—for example, my son would play with his Legos, and when it was time to clean up, he would look at me and say, 'I can't.' Well, I would get upset and tell him, 'Of course you can. Clean it up.' It became this horrendous situation. The psychologist explained to me that he really can't clean it up—that I needed to break things down: 'Pick up the blue Legos,' and when he finished that I'd say, 'Now pick up the red,' and so forth. I have used that in almost every aspect—cleaning his room, completing homework assignments. He doesn't say he can't; he does it in small steps, and it has been a godsend to know that."

When All Else Fails

1. Remember the "broken record" technique? This one may come in handy on many occasions: "I understand what you are saying, but I'm still concerned that. . . ."
2. Get a second opinion. This is a perfectly appropriate and medically recognized approach to handling uncertain situations and should be gladly agreed to by your child's physician. If she gets defensive or seems peeved, you may want more than just a second opinion. If she is agreeable and supportive of this approach, this bodes well for your partnership. For starters, ask her whom she would recommend. If that doesn't work, go back and try the suggestions above under the heading "Sources of Referrals to Good Doctors."
3. And, of course, there is always the last resort: speak with other parents to get information on other doctors in the area who really know the disorder and treatment.

Parents' Top Ten: How to Make Sure Your Child Gets the Best Possible Treatment

1. "Don't rely only on medication, and don't refuse to try it."
2. "Don't give up until you find the right combination of environment, medical, and therapy supports to help your child improve her functioning."
3. "Seek quality medical care. Ask the doctor for patient referrals—whom he or she has treated—so you can talk to them. Do not settle for what one doctor or therapist tells you. Always get a second opinion if you are unsure."
4. "Try various behavior modification–diet changes–lifestyle adjustments and decide what works for your child. Do not just give medicine as the doctor prescribes. Watch what works for your child and ask for med adjustments/changes if you think they are needed."
5. "I keep a running journal of my son's appetite, behaviors, etc., and give them to the doctor when we go in. He says it helps him immensely."
6. "The most important thing a parent can do is read, read, and read. Don't automatically take the word of physicians, psychologists, and other 'specialists.' It would be great if they were all well versed in ADHD and all had our best interests in mind when diagnosing and treating, but they do not. Many are not willing to make a diagnosis because of their biases. Others will diagnose and recommend unproven treatments and therapies that they most often provide and profit from. Reading information that comes from nonprofit organizations, such as CHADD, and books by reputable physicians that are known specialists in the field are important. Look for scientific studies, not just claims."
7. "We enlisted the support of our pediatrician to call and plug our request to be seen, and then we waited about four months for the evaluation. But without wherewithal, determination, money, insurance, and a little 'pushiness,' we would not have been seen."
8. "My single most important piece of advice to a new parent: You can be your child's number one advocate and the expert with regard to all facets of his or her life, but you must educate yourself, and you have to be comfortable with relying on the currently available medical and psychological information, as well as relying on your instincts, and feeling good about your decisions without second-guessing yourself all the time."
9. "Get a good doctor who knows his stuff, and find a medication that works for your child. It's the single best thing to do, and many parents don't understand medication issues: that if one doesn't work, move on to another. You need to stay positive about trying meds to help the child deal with it. You need a doctor who also understands the trials of medication issues and will manage meds well."
10. "Understand that there is no one doctor that seems to understand all the complexities of ADHD. The first psychiatrist we were referred to knew *nothing* about what drugs to prescribe. He prescribed a combination of drugs that caused a severe reaction. I wish/think someone should have told us that ADHD is seldom the sole issue you're going to have to deal with."

Making Your Healthcare Providers Work for You

Remember, the doctor is not the only person you have to deal with in getting the care your child needs. A receptionist may be the person actually responsible for making appointments, copying records, typing up reports, filing insurance claims, or giving you copies of billing statements. Whoever fills this role in your child's doctor's office is a key player, and you must pay just as much attention to this relationship (perhaps even more!) as you do to the relationship with the doctor. Remember our discussion of the go-to person at the clinic in Chapter 4. A receptionist who is looking out for you will be very effective in calling special requests to the doctor's attention, reminding her of a report or letter to write on your behalf, or to return your phone call. Likewise, some offices have a nurse or nurse practitioner who can handle critical aspects of your child's care: regular tracking of height and weight, pulse and blood pressure; providing educational materials; assisting you in putting a behavior program in place; or coordinating the treatment plan with the school. Find out the roles of the various staff in your doctor's office and learn how they can help. How do you do this? The simplest thing is to ask either the receptionist or the doctor. Then, remember that your relationship with these folks may be what helps you get what you need, when you need it, from the doctor. You are not there throughout the day to remind him of your requests, but they will be. They need to be on your team, too. Do not neglect them at holiday time, when cards and cookies are very much appreciated by these folks, who rarely get such nice treatment throughout the year.

Questions to Ask about Who Does What in Your Doctor's Office

The best approach here might be to ask the nurse or receptionist if you can come to the first appointment early to talk these things over—or in what other way you could familiarize yourself with the office routines and roles, with a minimum of inconvenience to everybody.

- Who sends and receives information from the child's school, such as reports, checklists, and so forth?
- Who types up the doctor's letters and reports? Who sends them off to the school?
- Who takes the child's height and weight, pulse, and blood pressure? Who draws blood when it is required?
- Who provides information on ADHD, its treatment, and any tools or toolkits?
- Who assists with putting together behavioral treatment plans?
- Who might attend the child's educational staffing meetings and IEPs, when such is required?
- Who prepares the billing statements and send forms to the insurance company?

- Who makes copies of records for you?
- Who makes appointments? Who schedules in an emergency, when such is needed?

EXERCISE 4

Evaluating and Improving Your Communication Style

Whether it's the doctor or therapist, a nurse, the receptionist, an office manager, or a social worker, effective communication is key to your partnership with these other members of your child's mental healthcare team. If the system doesn't seem to be working for you, start trying to fix the problem by evaluating your communication style and skills:

- Are you a passive communicator? If so, you tend to keep your feelings to yourself, which often results in your giving in to others out of a sense of inferiority. Ultimately, you allow others to decide on the services your child will receive.

- Are you an aggressive communicator? Do you attack the person rather than the problems? Is there a tinge of hostility in your approach? If so, you probably don't show respect *or* receive it—or the services your child needs.

- Are you an assertive communicator? Do you confront the problem instead of the person? If so, you voice your feelings, seeking to work toward goals and make your own choices.

    Obviously, being an assertive communicator is the most effective style, but it doesn't always come naturally. You may not even be fully aware of how you come across, because if you feel intimidated or anxious, your communication style may be expressed mainly through body language. Effective body language involves the following; practice on your family if you think your body language lacks these elements:

    Establish and maintain eye contact throughout the conversation.

    Direct your face and body toward the person and keep a straight posture.

    Incorporate facial expressions and normal hand gestures to represent your thoughts.

    Maintain your moderate tone and pitch.

    Remember, many doctors are not accustomed to assertive, capable, and inquiring parents. Even though things are changing, the "doctor knows best" approach is the way most of us were taught, instead of how to form true partnerships with parents. So be patient. Cut us a little slack. Maintain a pleasant demeanor and use the broken-record technique. The most important thing is that you feel increasingly comfortable with your knowledge of your child's needs (if you have been doing your homework), and with your abilities to advocate for them. You don't have to get upset or defensive, because, going back to my military analogies, you hold the high ground. In most cases, you can release the doctor from service, if need be, so there's no sense wasting too much energy on trying to move a heavy stone when you can just as easily go around it.

If you find you are almost always in conflict with your doctor, and you've already changed doctors several times, it might time to take a step back and ask yourself if your manner is more abrasive than you realize, especially if some honest self-examination tells you your body language could use some work. To get another view of where you might be going wrong and what you can do about it, consider role-playing your conversation(s) with the doctor and ask another parent for feedback. Ask your role-playing partner for advice on what you could change to avoid putting the doctor on the defensive, then practice communicating in that new way.

Once you feel comfortable with your new communication style, try it out on the doctor. When you do, rely on the broken-record technique while using your new body language. Avoid any hint of blaming ("You didn't . . . ," "You don't . . . ," "You won't . . ."), saying instead something more about your concerns and feelings: "I'm worried about the medication because . . . ," "What can we do to resolve . . . ?"

If this approach doesn't cool things off, go home and review the exchange. If you think it's at all possible that the communication problem lies with you, especially if it's body language, you might want to save your potentially difficult discussions with the doctor for the phone or delegate these negotiations to your child's other parent and see if that makes a difference.

If not, you have a pretty strong indication that the problem lies with the doctor. In that case, try another tack if you have reasons to want to stick with this doctor. Can you try to infer the way the doctor prefers to communicate and adapt to it? Can you try communicating through a staff member whenever possible? If all else fails, you may have found a somewhat old-fashioned, incorrigible doctor who has trouble forming a partnership, and you'll have to move on.

Making Your Insurance Plan Work for You

At risk of demonizing the insurance industry, these stories are probably all too familiar:

"Everywhere I turned I was blocked by our insurance plan, which didn't want to let us see a psychologist or use some of the newer, more expensive medications."

"Reimbursement has been extremely difficult. Our son's ADHD doctor will not accept insurance and makes us battle it out ourselves."

Many insurance companies and plans are a godsend to parents of a child with ADHD, but it's an inescapable fact that healthcare is becoming more and more expensive, and many parents are being forced to choose between soaring premiums and plummeting insurance coverage. And they still have to deal with the possibility that coverage will run out or be denied, or that they'll have to pay a lot out of pocket to use a provider they prefer:

> "For counseling our insurance has a $5 co-pay. This covers a limited number of sessions, so I'm unsure at this point what will happen once we've used up the allowed number of sessions. I'm hoping that they will continue coverage."

> "I switched coverage to be able to continue with the same therapist, but now have to pay a $300 deductible and fifty percent of the cost of each visit. I have cut back our appointments so I can afford to go, but I am not convinced the infrequent appointments are as productive or helpful to my children."

Obviously, knowing the ins and outs of the system is paramount, especially since mental healthcare coverage varies so widely.

What You Should Expect Your Insurance Plan to Do for You

First, you have to know what your plan covers, and this depends on many factors, such as whether you are part of a health maintenance organization (HMO), a preferred provider organization (PPO), a fee for service (FFS) arrangement, or some combination of these. The following chart compares the salient features of the major types of insurance plans. If you currently are covered under one of these but have other options through your employer, this chart may help you determine which is the best choice for you. The details of the particular plan will always, however, be the determining factor. For example, the HMO your employer offers may be the best choice if the PPO option includes very few of the types of practitioners you'll need

Comparing Types of Healthcare Coverage

Type of healthcare coverage	Costs to you	Your flexibility to choose doctors	Whom the doctor works for	Co-pay
HMO	Similar to PPO	Less	HMO	Little or none
PPO	Similar to HMO	Intermediate	Self, but via a contract to the PPO, chosen by you	Preset and limited to a certain amount by the PPO
FFS	Usually higher than HMO/PPO	Maximal	Self, but hired by you	Determined by the doctor, usually higher

for ADHD but the HMO is extensive, or if any of the plans will pose practical problems, like forcing you to travel a long way to get covered services. But the PPO may work best for you if the practitioners you favor are the same ones listed as "preferred" (and therefore covered at a higher percentage) by your plan.

In an HMO, all medical personnel are hired directly by the corporation. Examples of this type of healthcare system are Group Health, located mostly in the Pacific Northwest, and Kaiser Permanente, located mostly but not solely in California and Oregon. Such organizations usually cover everything you need, and the pediatrician or primary care provider technically can see you as often as it takes to get the job done. By and large, it should not cost you more to be seen on a more frequent basis (though such organizations often charge a very small fee per visit). This means that you should be able to get frequent monitoring for your child. And there is usually almost no paperwork, which is a great relief.

Challenges sometimes seen in such systems are that you can't easily see a specialist (such as a child psychiatrist) without first getting a referral from the primary care provider. In addition, your child sometimes won't get the same doctor for each visit, but instead sees whoever is available. This erodes good-quality care, which often depends on good doctor–patient relationships, so some HMOs are trying to let you keep the same doctor throughout, a much more preferable approach. And last, there are only so many doctors available. So, for example, if you can't form a good relationship with either of the two pediatricians in the HMO in your area, you are out of luck, because there are no other choices. And going to someone outside of the HMO means that you pay full freight.

There are various arrangements of PPOs, but they often boil down to this: Certain providers agree to a set fee for the services they provide, then when you see them via your insurance plan, you and your insurance plan get charged, no more, no less. You may have a fairly broad choice of doctors, but you usually will have to go to one doctor's office for your child's care, another office to see the psychologist or counselor, yet another office for any other type of specialist your child may need, and still another office site for your own care. Unlike the HMO, in a PPO arrangement, the providers work on their own, in their own locations. You may have to do all the paperwork for insurance reimbursement yourself, or sometimes the doctor's office will file all paperwork for you, asking only that you pay the agreed-upon difference. More hassles for you, but more options for choice.

The last arrangement, is called FFS, in which the doctor usually bills you directly, you pay the fees, then you submit paperwork back to your insurance company to get reimbursed. It is important to know what kind of services and how much (in frequency, as well as in dollars per visit) your insurance plan reimburses, however. Your pediatrician may charge $40 for a routine visit, but your insurance plan may be willing to pay only $25. The rest is up to you. Or in another common variant, your insurance plan may pay eighty percent of the costs of such visits but set a limit on the total number of visits. Or it may pay for a visit to treat your child's strep throat but refuse to pay for a visit for ADHD, claiming that the latter is a mental health condition and must be handled by a specialist. Often in such circumstances, your provider may then give you a list of mental health providers, and you call all of them, only to find that none has any openings, or that the list is outdated and most have either moved away or no longer work with your insurance company. So this is a tough area, in which you are going to need maximum moxie and not take no for an answer. Be forewarned, there may be lots of paperwork and time spent on hold on the phone, just to get what you need or be appropriately reimbursed with some of the more problematic companies. You'll want to take advantage of the sample appeal letter in Appendix II.

You have the right to expect from your insurance company a clear overall description of what your healthcare plan does and does not cover, including (1) any per visit charges, such as in an HMO; (2) amount of deductibles; (3) total amount of coverage for routine pediatric visits; (4) any limitations on number of visits; (5) any limitations on the *types* of visits allowed by your primary care provider (e.g., is an ADHD visit allowed?); and (6) information on how you can access specialists, such as mental health providers, which are often "carved out" of the overall plan and treated as a separate item. It is best to know all of this critical information up front, since a lot of reimbursement decisions by the company will hinge on these points. And finally, you have the right to expect interpretable billing statements that tell you what your plan did and did not reimburse for any visits where you paid out of pocket or the doctor's office billed the insurance plan directly.

Taking Charge: How to Get What You Need from Insurance Plans

Here are some ideas for dealing with various insurance problems.

What to Do When Coverage Is Unclear

If you don't know exactly what your company does and does not pay for in terms of your child's healthcare, you may find it in the small print in your insurance policy. If this is unclear, write a letter and request the needed information in writing from the company. While this is a bit of extra work, it's worth the effort. Before you write the letter, find out who and where the "Insurance Commissioner" is in your state, and be sure to copy that office at the bottom of the letter, as well as your employer or the "benefits manager" in your company, since employers often purchase the prepackaged types of plans you get offered. Each state has its own insurance department to oversee all types of insurance; check the list at *www.hiaa.org/consumer/state_ insurance.cfm*. In addition, free insurance counseling and advice (federally and state funded) is available in each state, accessed at *www.hiaa.org/consumer/insurance_ counsel.cfm*. And last, the Pharmaceutical Research and Manufacturers of America (PhRMA) offers an online directory of patient assistance programs (including no- or low-cost medications) run by over 40 of its member companies (*www.helpingpatients. org*).

A *caveat*: Watch out for requirements that many managed healthcare companies have for getting preauthorization for certain services. If you skip this step and use a service, such as a specialist, without going through your company, or without getting a referral from your primary care doctor, you may be liable for the costs. Your company should have all the rules available in printed form, and most of the time your insurance card will contain a reminder about preauthorization. Be sure you know the rules, and if you have any doubts, ask the company to specify the requirements for preauthorization.

Ideally, you will want to avoid any companies that cut you a bad deal, rather than find yourself stuck with one after the fact. If the choice is yours, the U.S. Agency for Healthcare Research and Quality provides additional guidance on choosing your health plan at *www.ahrq.gov/consumer/hlthpln1.htm*.

What to Do If the Plan's ADHD-Related Coverage Is Insufficient for Your Needs

Here's a common dilemma: "Some of the insurance plans that we have been on covered ADHD under mental health disorders, and the benefits were limited." Another parent concurred: "My medical plan is not unusual in that it places limits and maximums on 'mental and nervous conditions.' With weekly counseling, it doesn't take long to reach those limitations. The dollars that were previously budgeted for private education tuition are now being directed to these healthcare expenses." A third parent wanted to see global change in this area: "I wish that mental illness would be covered the same as physical illness and have written letters to legislatures at the prompting of CHADD and others. The responses from most legislatures seem to hinge on the fear of skyrocketing insurance costs to employers who may opt out of offering insurance coverage at all."

If your employer struck a raw deal for you months or years ago, you may have to work with the employer (or your employer's benefits manager) to make sure that the next time a healthcare plan is negotiated and purchased for employees, the plan more fully meets your needs. Often this is done as frequently as yearly, so your efforts here can make a difference pretty quickly.

If you're stuck with this raw deal for the foreseeable future, however, parents have a few ideas you may be able to use:

- "My employer offers only one type of insurance. Once the company denies something, I immediately write back and justify why it should be covered. I have failed only once, and that was for an 'experimental pediatric drug.' "
- "We switch insurance companies when we encounter this problem. Or I take my daughter in with another vague illness or for her allergies and get an ADHD prescription while I was there. That way the visit was covered under the medical insurance plan."
- "Our previous insurance company had a limit on the amount of psychiatric expenses they would pay in a year's time. In the beginning, both my son and I racked up large bills, and they covered only a fraction of them. I am still paying those bills. Since then, we have switched insurance companies, and they cover most of the expenses. However, the co-pay for my son's ADHD checkups at the doctor are $25 instead of $15. The insurance company's response is that ADHD is psychiatric and not medically related. So when I take him in for a cold, I try to get his meds filled to get the cheaper co-pay."

• "I take full advantage of a Flexible Spending Account for Medical Expenses through my husband's employer." The law allows this parent through his employer to set aside pretax (tax-free) income dollars in a separate account that is then used to pay medical expenses. Depending on your tax bracket, this may save you up to thirty percent on your medical bills. Check to see whether your company has this option available.

• Also consider "visit management." If things are just beginning, I usually like to see families I work with every two to four weeks. If things progress well, meaning that the family is able to put a behavior therapy plan into place and the medication is effective, I pretty quickly space visits out to once a month, then gradually to once every three months, but no less than that. If you can't afford visits as frequently as you or your doctor thinks are necessary, see if you can spread them out a bit more, thereby reducing the overall cost burdens to your pocketbook. Discuss this with your doctor, however, since frequent monitoring of medication and frequent doctor–teacher communication has been shown to yield maximal medication management and optimal outcomes.

What to Do When Claims Are Denied or Coverage Is Limited

"I have changed psychiatrists due to my frustration with the system," explained one parent. "My insurer was the biggest issue; they referred us to an adult neuro-psychiatrist who was not set up to deal with children. His results deemed my son 'too hyperactive to test.' I had to get my son retested a few times to make sure he had no learning problems that can frequently be associated with ADHD." Coverage can be denied or limited in many ways by your insurance company. Here are some suggestions for responding, so that you get what your child needs.

Use Your Contact at Your Insurance Company

As noted in Chapter 4, you need to groom your relationship with the person who processes your insurance claims. Often, for a given state or a given employer, there may be only a small handful of people you will have to deal with, but first you need to get their names. Develop this relation using the strategies outlined in Chapter 4. Explain your dilemma, listen carefully, and try to do all they suggest. Get the person's name, the *full* name, introduce yourself, and use the person's first name in the conversation. Personalize this contact; use humor and all of your charm. Then, when you mail in the claim form, address it "Attention: [First Name, Last Name]," attaching a special note thanking the person for the special help, perhaps even commenting on some memorable aspect of the conversation! Keep this person as your friend and contact. Most likely, you are going to need him or her over time.

Parents who cultivate these contacts might get the following kind of information: "Well, I am not supposed to say this, but tell your child's doctor to use the XYZ billing code, not the ABC billing code. Our company doesn't cover ABC as well as XYZ." You may also find that you can ask your contact information about which codes or types of claims are best covered.

Remember that the persons you have to deal with are real human beings, but sometimes you have to make them real to you and, perhaps even more important, make yourself real to them. Requests made personally and on the basis of a good relationship are always most effective, and anonymous written letters, follow-up letters, and phone requests, while necessary, are "next best" strategies.

Follow Up in Writing

When you don't get a response to your own request for information or additional coverage from your insurance plan—and this is good advice when there's no follow-up on clerical requests from your provider offices as well—such as a copy of a medical report, write again, with "SECOND REQUEST" at the top of the letter, perhaps with a special, personal copy ("cc") at the bottom to your friendly contact, noted earlier, or if things are really grim, to the person or persons, or state office with oversight authority in that area. This can be a strong step, so don't use this unless you really need to, are certain you're getting the run-around, or if you want to risk the relationship. But sometimes you may not be able to personalize/humanize the relationship (such as in the anonymous insurance company, where you can't get a good name or contact), and you might need to take this step.

Seek Support from Advocacy Groups

In all instances, there is somebody with extra clout or authority that you can bring into the loop, such as your company's plan administrator (call the personnel office if you don't know who this is) or the state's insurance watchdog agency. To find your state agency, go to *www.hiaa.org/consumer/state_insurance.cfm*. One helpful national resource is the National Health Law Program (*www.healthlaw.org/consumer.shtml*), which can provide additional information on your state's health insurance consumer protections. As a bonus, if you are now in the mood to switch plans, this site also provides information on choosing an appropriate health insurance plan and other tidbits. Remember, too, that there are many agencies whose principal mission is to protect your child's rights.

> "With our first insurance program we were resigned to only getting meds covered. Appointments were fifteen minutes long and occurred once every three months. It wasn't sufficient for the doctor to get to know Trina or be very involved in her care. . . . It was all about getting prescriptions refilled. Eventually we got another insurance program, but we had to fight for the services that I knew were available. I had to complain to the Center for Disability Law before we got a qualified therapist, respite services, and a case manager. Fortunately, I had some connections in the system, so eventually I was listened to."

Every state has a protection and advocacy system to advocate for the disabled, including people with ADHD. Protection and advocacy (P&A) systems in each state are federally funded to assist people with mental or developmental disabilities in understanding and asserting their rights. To contact your state's P&A, please visit the website of the national association at *www.napas.org*. Often, but not always, these agencies are private, nonprofit, and linked with or operated under the auspices of the state's legal aid organization, frequently designated by the governor of the state. They can provide an array of services and advice that may be of help to your child, including advocating for a child's rights to insurance coverage for ADHD. Other tools to assist you include the free online resource from the Commission on Mental and Physical Disability Law at *www.abanet.org/disability/lawpract.htm*. You may also find other agencies in your state on the Bazelon Center website's list of state advocacy links at *www.bazelon.org/links/states/index.htm*, as well as other national-level protection and advocacy groups at *www.bazelon.org/links/other.htm*.

Ask Your Doctor to Help

Sometimes you can ask your doctor to write a special letter making the case that a given treatment, such as a particular medication, is in fact needed, even though the company doesn't normally cover it. In most instances, exceptions are possible, since the company would put itself at medical–legal risk to deny something that your doctor in fact said is necessary. You will probably have to find out the details of where and whom to write, but most doctors will do this, particularly if you get them all the details.

Be prepared, however, for the possibility that this maneuver won't succeed. "We tried to have the insurance cover the name brand Adderall for my son," one father told me. "The doctor wrote a letter and made a follow-up call to the company. He was told that if he did not drop the issue, he would no longer be on the provider list. The insurance company refused, and we filed a complaint with the state insurance commissioner. We're waiting to see what's going to happen."

Appeal Any Adverse Decision

All health insurance companies have internal grievance and complaints procedures. If you have a complaint, ask your contact how to do it, and be sure to follow the company's procedures. If the company rules that it will not cover a given disorder, treatment, or provider, don't take no for an answer. For example, if the company wants you to use one of its approved providers, you may find out that none of these "approved" providers are available, that they all have six-month waiting lists, or that none has the necessary expertise. What to do? Write a letter of appeal about their decision or ruling, documenting the problem. Copy the letter to the state's insurance commissioner. Call the insurance company back and follow up, then send yet another letter. This will take time and effort, but it often works. And once you have beaten them into submission, it should not be necessary to do it every time. And remember to use your contacts at the insurance company! See Appendix H for a sample letter that you might use to appeal a decision.

Watch for Mistakes

Remember, too, that sometimes mistakes are made, by your insurance company, a healthcare provider, a billing clerk, or someone else. You could be charged for the difference between the insurance coverage paid to the doctor and the doctor's usual fee, even when the doctor has signed an agreement with your company to charge only a certain amount. Or you could be asked to pay at the time of service, even though your plan calls for you to pay only a co-pay. Most providers have to work with many different sets of rules and companies, and they can get just as confused as you. Or a claims processor at your insurance company could make a mistake; it happens all the time. So you have to take time to learn the rules and identify situations where you are not obligated to pay any additional fees, or at least, less than the bill you receive suggests. Remember to put it in writing and keep a copy for your files.

What to Do When the "System" Still Won't Pay Enough

Here are a few more ways to cover your expenses when insurance just doesn't do enough.

Ask Your Doctor for Medication Samples

How many samples your doctor has and how many you can expect (the doctor has other patients, too) is limited, of course: "Doctors will provide med samples, but only if I push for it," said one mother. "Sometimes, we get pills in larger doses and I have to cut them to the right dose with a pill cutter, because pills in larger doses are often cheaper." From another: "The psychiatrist has provided some free meds—usually enough to get us started or to help cover the times of transitioning doses, where you may be on a certain dose of only a week or so." Be aware, however, that each state has its own laws about the distribution of medications. In particular, for controlled substances like the stimulants often prescribed for ADHD, it is against the law for doctors to provide free samples.

Remember Public Insurance Programs

"Currently we have medication and treatment costs covered by Medicaid," one mother told me. "We are actually receiving better care and services there than we were in the private sector." Medicaid covers children below the poverty line and applies to approximately one-fourth of U.S. children and adolescents. Different provisions may also apply from state to state and sometimes even from city to city. "Because my income doesn't allow me to cover my children with insurance," said another mother, "they are covered under Medicaid. I have to say that I have *never* had any problems with any of his medical visits, psychologist visits, or medication being covered. They have always been great about covering everything." The Centers for Medicare and Medicaid Services (CMS) offers a wealth of information and a directory of state Medicaid offices on its website at *www.cms.gov/medicaid/default.asp.*

Another insurance program under which children with ADHD can be treated is CHIP, the Children's Health Insur-

---

Free or Low-Cost Medication Programs

Call the Pharmaceutical Research and Manufacturers of America publication order line (1-202-835-3450) to request their Patient Assistance Directory, or go online to *www.phrma.org.*

---

ance Program, which was passed into law during President Clinton's tenure to cover children of low-income families not covered by Medicaid (above the poverty line but still not insured). To learn more about your state's program, go to the CHIP website (*www.insurekidsnow.gov/states.htm*) or call 1-877-KIDS-NOW.

Explore No or Low-Cost Medication Options

Each of the major pharmaceutical companies has a no- or low-cost medication option for persons with instances of financial need and/or hardship. You must be assertive and on your toes to find out about the latest programs, however. One good strategy and resource is to call the Pharmaceutical Research and Manufacturers of America publication order line (see sidebar). Another strategy that can save you money is to request that your doctor get samples from the pharmaceutical company representative. This is an option that too often goes unexplored.

Another way to lower your medication costs is to ask your child's doctor to write prescriptions for generic rather than brand-name medications. Generic medications are often anywhere from twenty to forty percent cheaper, if they are available. A newly released drug is unlikely to have a generic form, unfortunately, since the company that first develops and markets a particular medication usually gets a patent and exclusive rights to produce and market the medication for seventeen years, at least in the United States.

Make sure your doctor knows the insurance plan's specific requirements to save time and unnecessary battles. In one case, not uncommon, a parent's insurance policy required the doctor to write "Medically Necessary" on every prescription, or the pharmacy was required to fill it with a generic.

Co-pays can often be reduced by asking for a ninety-day supply of medication, rather than just thirty days. Some mail-order companies sell ADHD medications in ninety-day supplies. Because it is still just a single prescription, the co-pay may be the same as the thirty-day prescription. Check around for this option, and talk to other parents for information about the latest companies that provide this option.

Ask Your Healthcare Provider for Reduced Rates

If you don't ask, the answer is no! Don't be shy about asking your child's physician or therapist about the possibility of reduced rates. Most professionals will accommodate a direct request or make some type of arrangement that can make the financial burden more tolerable. Ask about a "sliding scale" based on income or ability to pay. Private practitioners are likely to make special arrangements if asked directly; non-profit clinics usually have a variable fee (sliding scale) that is based on one's income. When in a financial pinch, sometimes parents find that they must change doctors or healthcare professionals, seeking out a nonprofit agency or clinic with explicit pro-visions for persons with financial needs.

Another way to get reduced rates is through a university or medical school clinic, if there is one near you. All hospital clinics will have this option, but again, if you don't ask, you won't learn about it. Sometimes a given doctor within a univer-sity clinic will have some authority to make recommendations for reduced rates or sliding scales. The hospital or clinic's business office will often have information.

When to Pay Out of Pocket for Specific Services?

Under some circumstances, you may decide it's worth it to pay out of pocket for a service you need, even though, in an ideal world, either your insurance company or perhaps the school would pay. For example, you might have trouble finding a cov-ered practitioner with the necessary expertise in ADHD, so you'll foot the bill your-self up front, afterward attempting to get the company to cover it. This can be a sen-sible tack, particularly if the financial sacrifice is modest. Battling the insurance companies takes energy, which is fine, if you have energy to spare. But if your finan-cial resources are less strapped than your emotional resources, you may want to get the best care you can now and save your energy for future battles to recoup your fi-nancial outlays.

Sometimes paying out of pocket for an expert evaluation can be a good way to make your case for coverage. If some medical expert you have retained does an eval-uation, then writes an appropriate letter of support for the kind of treatment your child needs, the letter may carry weight with your company as a valid statement of your child's medical needs, even if the recommendation goes against the company's routine policies regarding treatment.

Your Action Plan

Before we leave this section, take time to reexamine your plan. In particular, review your child's medical needs and see if they have been fully filled in. Are there needs for additional diagnosis, assessment, or treatment interventions? Fill them in now. Did any of the parents' comments lead you to rethink some of your assumptions? Did they give you some new ideas? Do you need to consider getting a different doctor? Did the information lead to possible changes in your short-term objectives? Pull out your plan and fill in any new areas you have thought of.

Also, at this time, create a new chart called your Intermediate-Term Action Plan (a blank is provided in Appendix F, p. 253). Use the same format as used for your short-term plan, but for this one, think about your child's needs from a some-what longer term perspective, namely, over the next twelve to eighteen months. For example, if a short-term objective for your child's social–emotional needs is to share toys and to have better temper control when he is with his playmates, an intermediate objective related to this short-term goal might be to develop a new friend with whom he gets along, sometime during the next year. Accomplishing the intermediate goal will require working on the short-term goal for a while, but it is important not to just have short-term goals. You want to know where your child is ultimately headed—in this case, better peer relations and one or two solid friendships. Look at the examples of needs in the left-hand column on the next page, but then fill in your own child's needs in the Intermediate Action Plan chart in Appendix F, including all five columns.

One parent said,

"Medicines become expensive, and therapies are expensive. It has tapped our resources, but we'd do it over if need be. In the end, we will do whatever necessary to help our daughter. With regard to insurance, we have received some misinformation about coverages, but have been persistent and pushed to have things covered that we were originally told wouldn't be. We've employed common sense and reasoned with our insurance provider, which has been willing to bend on occasion."

INTERMEDIATE-TERM ACTION PLAN

Your child's needs	Approaches How will the need(s) be addressed? Resources?	Who will do it? Who else will assist and be on your child's team?	When? What is the time frame for accomplishing specific tasks?	Outcomes Intermediate-term goals and objectives
Social–emotional needs 1. One or two stable friendships 2. Being good at a sport or other activity				
Medical needs 1. A doctor he likes and one I can trust 2. Medicine with fewer side effects				
Educational needs 1. Special education resource room and teacher				
Parent–family needs 1. I need better skills in using behavior therapy				

Six

GETTING THE BEST
FROM YOUR CHILD'S EDUCATION

"The lack of knowledge by the teachers regarding ADHD and their unwillingness to do anything special or make any special allowances for my child has been my biggest challenge."

"My son was diagnosed within the first six weeks of the first grade. However, because of his ADHD, he had missed out on all of the basic skills of reading in kindergarten. The hardest thing for me was realizing that it may take us years to get him caught up to the level of his peers and that it will be a struggle for him."

"Because the teachers at school lack understanding of ADHD, they most often expected that my son could control his own behavior—if only my son would 'just do' this or that or if at home we 'would do' this or that. The teachers would easily lose patience, which, of course, made situations much worse."

"The most important thing you can do is advocate for your child's needs. Teachers are good people, but the system doesn't always take into consideration the needs of its students. Teachers will advocate, but they don't follow your child through the system, you do. Ultimately, we as parents are responsible for the educational and social–emotional development of our kids."

If there is one key to success in getting the best for a son or daughter with ADHD, it is probably making the schools work for your child. School and schoolwork are where much of your child's self-esteem is built. For a child or teenager, succeeding at school is like you succeeding at your job. So how are you going to make that happen? As with making the healthcare system work for you, you're going to learn the territory, develop a plan, get help from others, and put your plan to work. The good news about the school system (at least the public schools) is that you have lots of help, *paid* help in fact. And if that weren't enough, the public schools are required by law to be helpful!

Making the School System Work for You

Trying to get what your child needs from school can, however, seem overwhelming. Your child has a disability that can make academic success difficult to achieve and social interaction a challenge. As you undoubtedly already know, if your child can't pay attention and is also disruptive in class due to hyperactivity, his teachers may feel he's only making their job harder: They can't get him to attend to his work, and on top of that he's distracting the *other* kids. Maybe the teachers are already unfavorably inclined toward him, and you all feel in a one-down position regarding these important figures in your child's life.

Then, there is the institution we call "school." Whether your child's school is public or private, it's sure to be bound by bureaucracy, and even the most well-endowed schools seem to have too few funds to answer all the needs of each individual student enrolled. Do you have to be the world's most persuasive, aggressive negotiator to get what your child needs at school? Not exactly, but there's no denying that you need both skill and knowledge. A little chutzpah never hurts either. And, finally, this, probably more than anywhere else, is where you need to be super organized. In this chapter, the short-term action plan you developed in Chapter 3 will begin to come to life as you add details concerning your child's educational needs and learn more about the *approaches* you can take, *from whom* you can expect help, and the *objectives* that you wish to accomplish (refer back to these three columns in your action plan).

What You Should Expect the School System to Do for You: Your Child's Rights under Federal Laws

First and foremost, remember that a cornerstone of our country's commitments to our children is to provide all of them a free and appropriate education, regardless of race, creed, color, gender, income status, religion, or disability. For kids like yours, these basic educational rights are established by two statutes: legislation passed in 1973 under the Civil Rights Act (Section 504) and more recent legislation called IDEA (Individuals with Disabilities Education Act). In depth, user-friendly summaries are available on the CHADD National Resource Center on ADHD website at *www.help4adhd.org/en/education/rights*. Links to the actual full legalese in all its glory can be found at *www.ericec.org/lawlink.html*.

Section 504 law provides that no one can be discriminated against on the basis of any of the factors mentioned earlier, including having a "disability." And because ADHD is a bona fide medical condition, and because it results in difficulties in the child's functioning, at no fault of his or her own, it is technically a "disability"—in this case, an educational disability.

Accommodations made to allow your child an appropriate education will vary from school to school and from state to state, but every school will have a list of them, known as the "504 plan"—a systematic strategy of procedures and accommo-

Should You Let the Schools Label Your Child?

"The hardest thing for me has been to accept the fact that I had to classify my son with a 'disorder,' " admitted one mother. Another stated, "The hardest thing has been the stigma associated with it and worrying that others would look at my son differently because of it." For many parents, seeking extra help at school means revealing to a wider world that their child has a disability and exposing the child further to the insensitivity of others. My response to those who ask themselves whether they should risk having their child labeled by the schools is, first, don't be put off by the term *disabled*. You may not—and need not—necessarily think of your child as "disabled," as you might more typically think of a child in a wheelchair. But schools are required to provide special accommodations for the child in a wheelchair, so he can get to classes and, in every way possible, participate fully in the school's educational activities. The same principle applies to ADHD. To the extent that your child's attentional difficulties make it hard for him to take full advantage of what the school has to offer educationally, the school must make accommodations to remove this potential barrier to learning. So a child may not need a wheelchair ramp, but the child with ADHD will need other accommodations, such as being placed near the front of the class, getting homework assignments in smaller chunks, and receiving extra reminders or monitoring to ensure that homework assignments are written down.

Also, keep in mind that the child who is struggling academically, who needs these services and who doesn't get them, is already labeled, not just by other kids ("loser," "goof-off," "not very smart," etc.) but even by himself ("I'm not very good at school," "Other kids are smarter than me"). So, from my point of view, the question facing you right now is not whether to label or not to label—that is happening already—but how to get your child the resources he needs to succeed, whether those resources come from general education programs, Section 504, or IDEA special education.

dations that can be made available to a child with ADHD. If you are not sure what these are, talk with your child's principal or call your local school district and ask to speak with the *special education coordinator* or *assistant superintendent for special education* (the title may vary from district to district). Ask that person for a listing or handout about the district's 504 plan provisions. And to see how it fits in, see Appendix A for a listing of 504 plan provisions.

The 504 plan provisions may be "just what the doctor ordered," but for some children with ADHD, they may not be quite enough to give that extra help needed to succeed. If your child's ADHD and related behavioral and emotional difficulties continue to greatly affect her school functioning despite good medical assistance and 504 plan-style accommodations, IDEA provisions will often apply. This law is also commonly known as "special education law" and requires more than simple accommodations. Instead, the law specifies that the school must provide rehabilitation, special services, and/or other related assistance to address any part of the disability that affects the child's education. For the blind child, that means the school must provide books in Braille or on tape. For the deaf child, it means the school must provide teachers who use sign language to teach. For the child with severe, unstable diabetes or asthma that often interrupts his school experience, it may require that the school provide the on-site services of a nurse to monitor the child's health status and to deliver medications when needed.

For the child with ADHD, special education services go beyond simple accommodation: The child with ADHD might need a somewhat smaller classroom, say with eight to twelve children and an extra aide, or one-on-one time with a teacher trained in special education techniques, a speech and language therapist, or "pull-out" classes (where the child is taken from the regular classroom setting for several hours a week and given more intensive educational services for one or more topics, or for behavioral assistance). Related one mother,

> "The biggest problem I have encountered is being blamed for my son's dependency on me. He lacks advocacy skills, and they say it's because I rescue him too much. Interestingly, since my son has been receiving the extra special education support at school, I have had to advocate for him much less! Since he's been getting the special education support, there are less meltdowns (*much* less), and I'm not in a position of having to advocate for him anymore. He is now in a better mental situation, so that I can help him with these skills. Before, he could not deal with it. The school wanted me to make him advocate for himself, but he could not have done it before special ed help."

> You have the right to expect that the school will respect your child's privacy and keep records confidential. *The school may not release them to anyone outside of the school system without your permission.*

Many other sources such as the CHADD Resource Center (*www.help4adhd.org/en/education*), the Technical Assistance Alliance for Parent Centers funded by the U.S. Department of Education (*www.taalliance.org*), states' protection and advocacy systems (*www.napas.org*), and others listed in Appendix D can give you all the details on your child's legal rights to an education and the legally mandated process for applying for special education or accommodations.

First, I present a brief summary of what the two laws provide:

- Eligibility for IDEA and an IEP authorizes that a child have a disability requiring special education services, while eligibility for Section 504 may occur when the child needs special education *or* any related services.
- Children who have less severe disabilities and need minimal accommoda-

tions, who are otherwise not eligible for IDEA, may be covered under Section 504.

- There are far fewer rules and regulations placed on the testing process in Section 504 than are outlined with IDEA for an IEP. Section 504 does not:

    Discuss the role of outside evaluations
    Limit the frequency of testing
    Require parental consent for testing

The Section 504 process does require that an evaluation be conducted before a child receives a 504 plan, and before any alterations are made to the proposed plan. In addition, because of the less strict safeguards provided by Section 504, you should be aware that certain situations may arise that the 504 plan won't cover. These may include a "stay-put" provision to keep your child in his current environment while any issues are being resolved or having the plan travel with the child through the grades.

So essentially, if your child's disability is considered to be on the milder side, she will probably qualify for classroom accommodations under Section 504. If she needs more help, she will probably receive special education under IDEA. However, both of these laws operate on the assumption that the child has some form of disability or impairment that is impeding her ability to have the same advantages of a free and public education as do children without disabilities. It doesn't mean that, as parents, we are entitled to whatever we want for our children—which is usually "the best" of whatever—but only those resources needed to level the playing field for the child with a disability.

What You Can Expect from Section 504

Section 504 specifically states that a local educational agency must offer a free suitable education in the least restrictive environment for children with handicaps, provided the impairment is documented and continuous. Children who fit into this category are those that have a physical or mental condition, including ADHD, that significantly limits at least one major life activity (such as learning). To provide a suitable education for the child, an accommodation plan can be developed for adjustments in a regular classroom. Some generalized accommodations are listed here, though specific adjustments should be individualized for each child. Additionally, you should remember to request that the decided accommodations be placed in writing and signed by all parties involved (school and parents).

Typical accommodations include the following:

- Modified homework assignments and testing.
- Supervision of homework assignments.
- Reduction in the amount of written work and/or extended deadline to complete any assignments.
- Access to a computer for written work, if easier.

- Alternate seating arrangements in the classroom (i.e., closer to teacher/blackboard).
- Use of helpful tools (calculator, tape recorder, electric spell checker).
- Continual progress reports assessing behavior and/or assignments.
- Behavioral intervention plan/social skills training.

If your child is deemed eligible under Section 504, the school district must develop a Section 504 plan, including possible accommodations, as described earlier. See Appendix A for an example of a checklist of potential 504 plan accommodations from the Kenosha Unified School District, Kenosha, Wisconsin, as well as a sample 504 plan for Isa Wild, age eight.

Please note that, unlike the IDEA law, regulations for Section 504 do not specify the frequency of review of the plan or the role of outside evaluations, nor do they require parental involvement. That does not slow you down, however, and you will need to be involved with every step of the process. The Department of Education is responsible for ensuring that states appropriately implement Section 504 in school settings supported by federal funds. However, if things do not go as you would have hoped or expected, you can file a complaint with the Disability Rights Section, Civil Rights Division of the U.S. Department of Justice at *www.usdoj.gov/crt/ada/adahom1.htm*.

What You Can Expect from IDEA Services

The federal IDEA requires that school districts provide special education services to students in a general education setting whenever possible, instead of in special, separate classes or schools. General education settings are also called the least restrictive environment (LRE) for students requiring special education services. I later list some of the *special education services* you can request if your child's evaluations document educational needs in various areas. All of these difficulties, and what will be done by the school system to address the difficulties, are detailed in a document called an Individualized Education Plan (IEP), which is basically a planning document, much like your action plan, except this one is required by law. If your child qualifies for special education services, you will be asked to participate in developing his or her IEP. See Appendix A (and other sources suggested earlier) for details on this process.

IDEA Services Provided within the General Education Setting

Supplementary Aids and Services

Children can receive aids and services based on recommendations from various evaluators, including occupational therapists and psychological, educational, or school-based teams. These services include the following:

- Varied instructional practices—cross-age tutoring and peer partnerships
- Behavior intervention plans

- Instructional adaptations—changing the pace or sequence used to present information
- Curriculum accommodations—audiotapes, calculators, word processors, and changes in the mode of presentations to use more picture symbols or overheads with key points
- Individualized supports—rephrasing of questions and instructions, allowance for additional transition time between classes, main idea summaries, highlighted reading materials, and organizational aides

If a school is limited in its ability to ensure the provision of these services in a general education setting, special education teacher support staff may be necessary to work with the general education teachers.

School-Based Counseling

One-on-one counseling in the school once or twice a week and/or counseling in small groups of three-on-one or five-on-one once or twice a week is based on the recommendation of the psychiatrist, therapist, or the school/district psychologist. Services are usually provided by the school psychologist, social worker, or guidance counselor.

Speech and Language Services

Based on the recommendation of a speech pathologist, services are given to help students with reading, writing, and speech. Services can be provided in the classroom, in small groups, or outside of the classroom one-on-one. Services are provided by a speech pathologist.

Resource Room Services

Based on the recommendation of the education evaluator, these services are given to help students with reading or math. Services are usually provided in a separate classroom in small groups of three-on-one or five-on-one. Services are provided by a special education teacher.

Test Modifications

These are changes in testing procedures or formats, which provide opportunities for students with special needs to demonstrate their knowledge and abilities on standardized tests. Modifications are based on the attention, processing, and learning deficits of a child and the recommendations of one or more of the evaluators. Testing modifications include tests given individually or in a small group in a separate location, or in a location with minimal distraction. Extended time, specified duration of testing time without breaks, directions read and reread aloud, answers recorded by any means necessary, use of calculators, and use of markers for tracking are also possible options.

One-on-One Service Providers

Other services are available on a one-on-one basis, such as *Crisis Management services*, which are considered when a child's placement has been found to be appropriate but the child's pattern of behavior is so acute that a paraprofessional is necessary; *Awaiting Placement services*, which are used until a child receives placement in a more restrictive education setting, such as a day treatment program; and *Transportation services*, considered for students who already receive transportation services but exhibit a pattern of behavior that is hazardous and beyond the norm of other students being transported.

Special Education Teacher Support Services

A variety of special education teacher supports are sometimes provided, including both direct instructional support by a special education teacher in a general education setting and consultation services by a special education teacher to the general education teacher to assist in the use of appropriate strategies to instruct a student in his or her regular classroom. If your child is eligible for these services, you should check with your local city, county, or district to determine what is available, because these services can be provided several times a week and for different lengths of time during the school day. All services must be specified on the IEP, including how much time the teacher is going to spend directly and indirectly with the student, as well as where and when they are going to do this work.

Collaborative Team Teaching

Another integrated approach in which a special education teacher and a general education teacher provide full-time instruction to a class of students, which includes a group of students with disabilities, is usually provided full time but can be provided in a subject area in a middle school or high school.

IDEA Services Provided within the Special Education Setting

If the needs of your child are great, services in a general education setting may not be enough to foster improvement in behavior, attention, or learning areas. It may also be necessary to consider special education programs if the child is nearing a transition to middle or high school and you wish to get him as much help as possible before that transition year approaches. You may also consider placing a child in a special education program, because all of the services delivered at different times by different providers are confusing or distracting. These include specialized classrooms, with changes in the teacher–student ratio, either fifteen-on-one, twelve-on-one, or six-on-one, with or without any of the other services noted earlier. In addition, emergency education services and transition education services can be made available to qualified students.

Caution: Anticipate Roadblocks Ahead

"We had to file a grievance with the school district because they would not offer services to our child under OHI (Other Health Impaired). Even when this school district did finally give in, it was the last week of school and we had experienced the worst year of school yet. We then transferred this OHI back to our home state, where his IEP was modified. All that the first school offered was content mastery and did not address his specific problems at all per the special ed law."

"Because of the teachers' lack of understanding of ADHD, they would blame my son for his behavior and hold him responsible for things he could not control. This was a travesty of justice for him. Also, I had him tested in school three times over five years. The first two times, they refused him extra help. It wasn't until this year (sixth grade) that we ended up with a teacher who had a base understanding of ADHD and recognized that my son's challenges were a result of ADHD. Because of her support and request for special ed help, he now receives the extra support needed. The special ed teacher says she wishes she 'would have gotten him two years ago!' "

Taking Charge: How to Get What You Need from the School

As you are finding out, as parents, we often find ourselves automatically placed in the role of being advocates for our child's education, and we may not have sufficient information about appropriate laws and available services. To aid those of us in this position, most school districts and state education offices have developed materials for parents to become better informed and knowledgeable about these services and how to access them. Also, parent support and education programs have developed around the country to assist parents in being informed advocates for their child's education. Organizations such as CHADD and the Learning Disabilities Association of America (see Appendix B) provide phone consultation, written information, and informative workshops. This whole school thing is a maze, so it is a good idea to have someone walk you through it (like an experienced parent who has done it before!), perhaps accompanying you to the school as you begin to learn more about what is needed and what you can do for your child.

The process of requesting and obtaining special education services for a child may differ slightly from state to state, but there are some general guiding principles. Every state has laws to define and protect the rights of parents in special education processes. To find out about those in your state, you can link to your specific state's Parent–Teacher Association (PTA) via *www.pta.org/index.asp*, find other agencies in your state on the Bazelon Center list of state advocacy links at *www.bazelon.org/ links/states/index.htm*, or go to the website of all states' Parent Training and Information Centers and Community Parent Resource Centers, federally funded to serve families of children and young adults with all disabilities from birth to age twenty-two. Later I give you the benefit of other parents' experiences in navigating this maze.

Taking the First Steps: What to Do If You Think Your Child Needs Special or Additional Educational Services

No matter where you live, the process of obtaining special services usually begins with either you or the teacher. It's not uncommon for the teacher to be the first one to spot a problem with a child's academic performance. In fact, it may be the teacher's desire to have your child evaluated that first alerts you to the possibility that your child has ADHD (and/or a learning disability or other problem). But since you're reading a book for parents of kids with ADHD, let's assume you already know your child has the disorder and now pursue getting the child whatever school help he needs. These are some of the initial actions that other parents and I have found helpful:

• If you haven't done your action plan yet, tut tut! You can't skip this step, or you'll pay a price later. Take some time away from home and work activities to make a list of what you think your child needs. Your gut instincts are critical here. What do you think would help him achieve his potential in the classroom? Would tutoring or extra one-on-one time with a special education teacher possibly be helpful? Assistance in math or reading? Being able to work on computer instead of by hand? Being changed to another class or another teacher? Thinking ahead this way will save valuable time and inject your well-informed opinions about what's best for your own child into the plan right from the start. Go to Appendix F and use the chart on page 252 to identify what you want to help your child with and which accommodations can do that.

• If your child is in elementary school, make an appointment to talk with the classroom teacher to express concerns and develop a course of action together. Don't make the mistake of skipping over the teacher and requesting an appointment with the principal. The teacher will play a key role in both planning and implementing any accommodations your child gets, so it's critical to forge an alliance with her right now.

• In middle or high school, make an appointment with the teacher responsible for the subject that is most problematic and devise a course of action together. Also, you might talk with the child's homeroom teacher or the school counselor assigned your child.

• If the teacher is not responsive to expressed concerns and you have tried everything else (I later discuss developing a working relationship with the teacher), you might need to contact the principal directly.

• In most localities, the principal may make referrals to a special team in the school, sometimes called the School Support Team, Pupil Support Team, or Student Support Team (the name varies from district to district) to work out an intermediate plan of action that may include more observation, evaluation, some services for a temporary period, and so forth. After some specified period of time, the team may make a referral to special education services for a special educational testing and evaluation. In some schools, these teams do not exist, but they will be available *by law* at least in the district. In such cases, you will have to work directly with the district's director of special education or with whomever the principal refers you. Go in well prepared with your knowledge of the IDEA and Section 504 laws, so that you are not caught flat-footed—"I am so sorry, Mrs. Smith: we don't have any testing slots until next school year." You might even come in prepared with an independent evaluation that you have paid for, in order to get all your ducks lined up. Or bring along an experienced parent advocate who has done this before.

• In most cases, it is these evaluations that will determine whether your child qualifies for services at all and, if so, under Section 504 or IDEA. But keep in mind that since Section 504 is a civil rights law, you can contact either the local school district or your regional Office of Civil Rights of the U.S. Department of Education to ask questions about how this law might be applicable to your child. Check your phone book under the U.S. Department of Education for the address and phone number of the office closest to you, or go to *www.ed.gov* on the Internet. As of the writing of this book, that site contained a highly informative piece called "Protecting Students with Disabilities: Frequently Asked Questions about Section 504 and the Education of Children with Disabilities" that you might want to read before talking to the school district. Once you do decide to talk to the local school district, however, first go to your child's teacher and/or school administrators to find out how to contact the district's 504 plan coordinators, since each school district handles 504 plans differently.

• To make sure you fully understand your district's 504 plan procedures (they vary), ask for a copy of your district's Policies and Procedures on Section 504. This document may be referred to by various names, including Procedural Safeguards, Parental Rights, or something similar. This document will inform you of your and the school's rights and responsibilities in getting your child the accommodations he may need.

• If you decide to request a 504 plan, be sure to put your request in writing. You should date and sign a letter that explains the purpose of the request by indicating where the concerns and problem areas lie. Some schools have forms for these "request for referral" letters. Remember to make a copy (for your files!) and if possible, *personally* give the original to your child's school for its records. Upon delivery, the school is required to begin an evaluation process following strict and clearly defined guidelines. Remember, to receive services under Section 504, a child must first be determined to have a disability that substantially limits one or more major life functions, including education, learning, and behavior. Only the school can determine whether your child qualifies for accommodations. You can assist this process if you have a letter from your child's doctor or therapist that is officially rendered as his or her professional opinion.

• *Terrific tip from parents:* "Right at the start of this process, ask for a complete listing of the kinds of resources the school has available, so you know what's within reach—and what you may have to pull a lot of additional strings to get. You have a right to this information, and having it early will give you a valuable heads-up."

Participating in the All-Important Evaluations

Once you've contacted the school with your concerns, the school may be able to create a temporary action or intervention plan for your child, while the referral to the team responsible for special education in the school is being made, if school personnel believe the problem is urgent. This referral will start a series of evaluations and tests requiring your written consent. Their job is to determine your child's strengths, where the difficulties lie, what services your child needs, and what modifications are required to ensure that he reaches his academic potential. *In the event that the school denies testing, under law, you have the right to appeal the decision.* I'll talk about that later in this chapter. The following are components of the evaluation process:

- *Social history.* All evaluations begin with meeting the parents to document the family structure, the home environment, and the child's physical development, emotional history, school history, social life, hobbies, interests, challenges, and so forth.
- *Psychological evaluation.* A comprehensive psychological evaluation will be done unless a recent evaluation was done privately to submit to the school psychologist. This evaluation includes several different tests that measure intelligence, academic achievement levels, perceptual and language processing, and ability to complete tasks within a certain time frame. Although it provides a lot of information, if ADHD or learning problems are present, other tests are necessary, such as educational achievement tests, language/perceptual tests, or neuropsychologic tests (see below). In most states, a comprehensive psychological evaluation is good for three years and will not be redone within one year. The school district may or may not allow these tests to be done by an outside evaluator, but if you have one done and it verifies the child's level of needs, I have never seen an instance where it was disputed by the school district, even though the district still did its own evaluation.
- *Psychiatric or neurological evaluations.* Because your child has ADHD, an evaluation from a psychiatrist or a neurologist will be necessary. A private psychiatrist may perform this evaluation, or the school system can refer you to an appropriate doctor. This evaluation will include recommendations that may consist of medications, therapy, counseling, and suggestions for the school environment, such as time-out breaks during the school day. Remember to get copies of all of test and evaluation results in writing for your records! This evaluation must be done by an MD. If you are already working with one, so much the better. Ask to review the letter before it is delivered, so that you don't get any surprises and can be sure it helps your child's case.
- *Education evaluation.* It is usually best for the school system to perform this battery of tests, which includes spelling, decoding, writing, reading, comprehension, and arithmetic and mathematical word problems, if possible, though sometimes you

may have to have it done by an outside evaluation team that you hire to get the school moving and to "prove" that your child has significant needs for which the school should provide services.

• *Other evaluations.* If your child has problems with spelling, reading, writing, or arithmetic, separate tests may be given by language or perceptual specialists. There may be problems processing language or a problem following words and numbers on a page. A speech and language or perceptual evaluation gives this type of information and determines whether additional services are necessary, and if so, what type of services are needed and how often they should be given.

• *Terrific tip from parents:* You have a right to copies of all of the results of the tests and evaluations the school does, so ask for them. Read them and ask your school contact who did the evaluation about any aspects of the evaluations that you don't understand or don't agree with.

• *Another terrific tip from parents:* If you have the financial and other resources to be able to do this, go out and obtain your own psychological, psychiatric, or educational evaluations if you have any concern that the school's evaluations won't be accurate, comprehensive enough, or rendered quickly. Very commonly, schools get backed up in terms of keeping up with the testing and evaluations they must do for children with potential special education needs. Also, remember, school testing personnel work for the school, and it can be hard for an evaluator employed by the school to press the school—his employer—to provide resources he knows the school lacks. Who wants to muddy the water he has to drink in? As I mentioned earlier, your own independent evaluations may give you a lot of leverage that you may not get if you rely only on the school's evaluation resources.

Getting an independent evaluation can be costly, and it may not be covered unless the doctor has ordered it for some justifiable medical (vs. educational) purpose. But if it becomes clear that the school system is not going to evaluate your child appropriately, it can be well worth the expense, as was the case for this family:

"My son struggled from the first day in school. He was kept back in kindergarten for 'developmental' reasons. In first grade, I requested that he be tested, because I suspected a learning disability. They wouldn't do any testing that year. In second grade, his teacher agreed with me, and he was tested by the school psychologist. After the testing, she told me he would do better in a regular classroom instead of going to a 'special' room for help. She said his self-esteem would suffer if he were pulled out of the regular class. She recommended counseling and tutoring. By the middle of third grade, my son was being treated for depression. The school system continued to say he just needed counseling. The social worker told me all the counseling in the world would not help if he continued to go to school every day and struggled. I agreed with her but couldn't get any support from the school. He had four tutors and two counselors for two years. In fifth grade, we were finally blessed with a teacher who recognized that he was struggling. She was a former LD [learning disabilities] teacher and suggested we have testing done. We went outside the school system and took the results back to the school. They then placed him in special ed under OHI for ADHD."

Sometimes the school system will have to pay for the outside evaluation, as this parent attests: "We have had the school pay for better testing and some extended therapy and specialists attending IEP meetings." In my experience, however, this level of success happens only when you have some legal leverage exerted by a lawyer you have retained.

• Outside evaluations usually come with letters or statements from the evaluators to the school indicating the types of educational resources your child may need. Likewise, you may have medical reports and psychiatric or psychological evaluations that will help school personnel make resource decisions about your child. Provide all of these to the school, with a cover letter from you, before the school evaluation begins, if you already have them, and as soon thereafter as possible if you don't.

• *One more terrific tip from parents:* Question any evaluation that doesn't seem comprehensive enough to identify problems you know your child has:

> "Initially, our son was not identified as having needs through our district's Early Childhood screening. The testing situation did not allow for easy identification of children with social–emotional needs. Our son is bright, with a strong vocabulary. That fooled them. I knew better, but I wanted to believe they were right. It took another couple of years before we actually got the help we needed. Once he was identified within the system at the kindergarten level, things improved for all of us."

• A caveat from one parent:

> "I made the mistake of having my son tested solely by a referral of the parochial school. A few years later, while being tested by a much respected physician in this particular field, we discovered that the first testing was performed by someone who was not respected at all within this field. I placed my faith in someone recommended through the church/school community, only to find out, much later, that the person was not qualified. The best advice has come through our pediatrician, psychiatrist, and counselor."

Evaluating the Evaluation and Developing the IEP

A team of qualified school professionals will review the completed evaluation and determine if your child meets the eligibility criteria. You will then be notified in writing. If she does not meet eligibility criteria, you can appeal this decision. If she does meet criteria, the next step is that you will be invited to a meeting, where an IEP will be created with your input and assistance. By law, you are an equal member of the team. The entire IEP process, from the initial meeting to the evaluation, to the actual IEP meeting, is highly regulated, with specified timetables along the way as to how long each part of the process may take.

As you and school professionals work together in the meeting, the IEP will list your child's needs, as well as goals he is expected to achieve by the end of one year. The team determines what services are needed for your child to meet the goals, where, whom they will be administered by, and with what frequency they will be delivered. You can agree or disagree with the final IEP recommendations but, ideally, you and the rest of the team want to come together to reach agreement on the final plan. If you agree, you indicate that and sign the IEP, which proceeds as outlined. But if you disagree, the law stipulates that you are entitled to "due process." The law also requires that the team meet at least once a year to review progress, and/or in the event the IEP needs to be changed, based on your child's changing needs.

Due process protects the rights of the parents and child. In the event you and the school district cannot agree about your child's needs and the school services required, a hearing is scheduled with an impartial mediator. Each side presents its arguments and evidence, and the hearing officer makes a final determination about what the educational program should be, based on the provisions of IDEA law. School districts are required to give you a copy of the special education procedural safeguards when an evaluation is first scheduled and each time an IEP meeting is held.

Assessing the IEP: Will the Plan Serve Your Child Optimally?

• *Don't settle for less when more is needed.* Now you have some knowledge of how to obtain school resources, and you may feel prepared to ask for what your child needs. Be forewarned that at some point you are likely to hear something like this: "We can't give everyone what your asking; we'd go broke. And there would be nothing left for other parents' children." This is an easy trap to fall into: No one wants to think that getting what his own child needs means depriving another child. But in fact, federal law stipulates that certain requirements be fulfilled for children with disabilities. Sure, schools are underfunded. But how are they ever going to get sufficient funding if parents don't stand up for their children's needs and rights?

So instead of feeling like you are asking too much, think of it this way: By advocating for your child, and pressing for additional resources when needed, you are helping the teachers, principals, and administration demonstrate that their students have needs that the state legislatures must support. Your clearly articulating your child's needs gives the superintendent more ammo when she tries to justify the yearly budget request. And as more and more parents like you stand up for their children, all children will be better served. So don't back off.

• *You don't have to say yes to whatever is offered.* Many times, once school personnel figure out that you are knowledgeable and effective in pursuing the necessary resources to help your child, you may be offered something and told "this is all there is." Well, if that is true, and it is not appropriate or sufficient for your child, just say no. You have the right to say no. If you do, the due process procedure will kick in. More about that later.

• *Terrific tip from parents.* Remember, when you go into an IEP meeting, if you don't take someone with you who is on your side, you'll be double- or triple-teamed. If you haven't gone to an IEP meeting before, take a friend along who has been there, seen it, and done it—someone big and tough, who can help you stick up for your child's needs. If you can afford it, even better, retain an experienced special education/disability rights lawyer. Regardless, if you are uncertain of anything, don't sign, and don't agree until you can go home, think about it, and talk with others, if need be. To obtain legal representation, contact the protection and advocacy system in your state via the national association (*www.napas.org*). Alternatively, you might contact the Commission on Mental and Physical Disability Law at *www. abanet.org/disability/lawpract.htm*. You may also find other agencies in your state on the Bazelon Center website's *list of state advocacy links* at *www.bazelon.org/links/states/ index.htm*.

• *Terrific tip from parents:* Once you get the proposed IEP from the team assigned to your child, and after you read these materials and factor them into your action plan, remember to file them! You are likely to need them later. In the concise words of one parent: "DOCUMENT EVERYTHING!"

Appealing Decisions

When you don't want to accept what is offered in your child's proposed IEP, you have at your disposal an appeal process ("due process") established by law. The school system must set up the process at no cost to you, which can be an expensive proposition for the school district. Therefore, at least in my experience, it is often easier for the district to give in and provide a resource requested by the parent than to go through the cumbersome legal process. Here are some tips from me and from other parents about how to make the most of the process:

• *To make your case, you may have to get an outside medical opinion about your child's special needs.* If the expense seems disproportionate, remember that this upfront expense may save you a bundle of money in the long run, once the school system begins to support what your child needs rather than forcing you to try to pay for all such services on your own.

• *Consider compromise.* You don't need enemies, particularly enemies who spend the day with your child, five days a week. For example, you might agree to revisit a currently denied service at the next IEP meeting. So you put in writing, if your child doesn't make such-and-such progress, then the following additional resources will be provided.

• *Be polite, be concerned, be understanding, but be firm.* The law specifies that children with specific disabilities, including ADHD, are entitled to the kinds of resources they will need to give them a good opportunity for educational success. If you believe that something denied in the IEP is critical, stand by your convictions. Said one parent: "My child still has the occasional 'slip' at school, but I have her IEP narrowed down to where it specifically spells out that they must contact me promptly. The school prefers a very 'broad' and vague IEP, but I simply requested a very specific one, with well-defined goals and objectives, and I refused to sign it until it was more specific, like I had requested."

• *When you feel like you've hit a dead end, don't give up:* "I ended up calling the Superintendent of the School Board and getting her out of the shower to get results for my son," said one parent.

Once the Plan Is in Place: What to Do When Things Go Wrong

Parents often feel as if their job is done once an IEP or Section 504 plan is finally in place. Naturally, though, your relationship with your child's school is ongoing. What do you do when problems arise? What if your child hates school and says she doesn't want to go back? Or your school says your child can't come back until he is "cleared" by the doctor or is put on medicine? The following tips should prove useful:

- Speak candidly and confidentially to the principal; ask for his advice. Asking for help and putting others in a position to help you, rather than leaving them to feel that you are demanding something of them, is often a good strategy.
- Get a second opinion, with an MD backup letter or phone call.
- Whom do you know on the school board? Talk with them.
- There's strength in numbers. Find out about good strategies from PTA or local parent groups such as CHADD and NAMI. What have other experienced parents done that has worked?
- Band together to present concerns to the principal.
- Go to the superintendent and request alternative arrangements.
- Last resorts: Pull out the big guns: a letter from your lawyer.
- Sometimes the battle isn't worth it. Is there another school around that you can transfer your child to? See the following sidebar for more on the pros and cons of moving to get your child into a better school.

Changing Schools: The Pros and Cons

Sometimes you just can't get what is needed in your current system, and tough decisions may be needed. Here's how other parents have made them:

"We had to give up the opportunity to buy an inexpensive house in the country to keep her in a urban school district with services. And we had to make sacrifices to buy a house in that district to keep her at that school."

"My son is not dumb. I can help him study for a test and he *knows* the material. But put the test in front of him and he will fail it. Finally I pulled him out of school at the second semester of his freshman year. I have been home-schooling him. This has been a challenge for both of us, since I am a single mom and I work full time. We do most of the work in the evenings, when I am home and can supervise. It has been a good experience for him, but I think he will be going back to school for his sophomore year."

Public versus Private?

Public and private schools vary, and one is not invariably better than another, as these parents' comments attest: *(cont.)*

"I had to make huge changes. I took him out of a private school and placed him in public school with many supports; a huge improvement took place this year. It was difficult to do, but it has paid off beautifully."

"I have not even attempted to put our son in public school. His private school first-grade teacher told us he didn't have ADHD, that he was just immature and should repeat the first grade. We switched him to a school for kids with ADHD, and by the end of that year, he tested at the sixth-grade level for math."

"We are planning to move this summer and chose a city based on not only our work but also whether there was a private school that could accommodate our son's needs."

"After two years of taking every kind of academic and psychological test and still seeing my daughter fail in school, I had to convince her that the heavy academic private school she was in was not right for her and take her away from her friends (at age ten) to enter a new school that could meet her needs better. We cried together every day for two weeks making that decision, saying good-bye to old friends and teachers who meant well. She trusted me enough to follow my guidance on this issue of switching schools, though it was her ultimate choice where to go. We began the school year (sixth grade) filled with anxiety and hope.

"With the proper environment, she has blossomed, grown, and is succeeding in most areas in school. She is working to her full potential, and she *knows* it. Hardly a day goes by that she doesn't thank me for putting her in her new school, which she doesn't want to miss, even over the holidays. Her self-esteem has mushroomed. Her unique talents are showing more each day. And she has a reputation for being a very caring student, especially toward those who struggle. Her musical and dramatic talents are being used, and she just shines. I would never have guessed I would be writing these words down, but her Dad and I are both very happy for her and proud."

"I elected to put my daughter in private school, where there are smaller classes and more individualized attention, and it as been very successful for her. She has gone from failing over half of her classes to being one grade off from the A/B honor roll."

"Since the local schools had a weak reputation for handling learning disabilities (and are severely overcrowded), we applied to several boarding schools that we felt could address both his giftedness and his LD. The first thing the school did right was to place him in all honors classes, and they have continued to recognize and challenge him academically. Second, the boarding environment has been very good for his social skills. Third, the psychologist and physician work with the school on counseling and medication management. We will see on the ultimate result, but the change has been very healthy."

"We were living in Los Angeles four years ago, when it became apparent to me that our kids could not get an appropriate education there. It wasn't that they didn't want to follow 504, but that there was no money and no teachers or resources to provide it. So we moved to an area where the highest amount per student was spent on education—the Midwest. Our other choice was back where we are from, to New York State, but Illinois had a much better IEP program in place, and the school district we are in utilizes every resource around! It's been a good experience, and we are glad we chose this school district after our exhaustive search."

EXERCISE 1

How to Get Your Child's Principal to Offer You Alternative Arrangements and Additional Resources When He Doesn't Think There Are Any

In each instance, consider what the principal says and what you might say that is an appropriately assertive response. Say your part out loud in front of a mirror.

PRINCIPAL: I am so sorry. We just don't have anything we can offer Joey at this point.

YOU: I'm sorry that resources are so tight. But we really need to find a solution to these issues. Joey has really been struggling, and we're going to lose him if we don't take action now.

PRINCIPAL: I know it's hard for you and Joey to wait, but there is really nothing we can do at this point. We are late in the school year, and all of our resources are committed.

YOU: This must be putting you in a difficult spot, I know. But I am not comfortable waiting any longer. Joey has fallen behind, and things are getting worse. We just have to do something. What would you suggest?

PRINCIPAL: Listen, I have a meeting I have to get to. I'll get back to you next week.

YOU: I know you must be terribly busy, and I wish I didn't have to take up so much of your time. But we do need a plan and some options that really are going to help him. Would it help if I had Joey's doctor call you? He has seen Joey and feels that additional resources are needed.

PRINCIPAL: I have to go. How about if I call you?

YOU: We've been waiting for some time, and you and I spoke about this several weeks ago. Should I call you at home tonight? We do need to get this resolved.

PRINCIPAL: OK, tell you what. See Mrs. Smith. Come in this Thursday afternoon, and we'll see what we can get going.

YOU: Thank you so much. I know how many pressures you are under, so I especially appreciate it.

Notice how you didn't give up. Notice also that you kept on your point, even after the principal had all kinds of reasonable delays. Also notice how you used the word *we*. And notice how you kept an understanding attitude toward the principal's dilemmas and scarce resources. These are all important aspects of keeping this a win–win situation. In other words, she has to feel good about helping you out, rather than feeling that she has lost a battle with you.

Terrific Tips from Parents:
How to Cultivate a Good Working Relationship with the School

When things go wrong, you're much more likely to get them going right again quickly when you've laid the groundwork for a fruitful alliance with your child's school. Here's what parents say has worked for them:

• *It all starts with good relationships with school staff.* In most cases, the people you have to deal with are just like you: They want to do a good job, they want to feel appreciated, and they usually give it their best. So if they feel under attack, they will revert to a defensive position and feel justified in fending you and your requests off as "unreasonable." Remember, a drop of honey usually gets you more than a gallon of gall. Go back to Chapter 4 for some suggestions for forming good partnerships with those critical contacts at the school.

• *Understand the school system's limitations.* It's important to convey understanding and empathy about the difficult spot school personnel often find themselves in: They have a difficult job, they are underpaid doing it, and they get too few resources to do a good job. When you press for additional assistance for your child, you may not be making their day any easier. So look for ways to avoid "I win, you lose" interactions. Whenever possible, create "win–win" strategies—for example, where you obtain the necessary additional resources you need for your child, but where you also get to thank school personnel for their understanding, their willingness to help your child, their going the extra mile, and so forth.

EXERCISE 2

Alternative Dialogues

How you say what you mean *does* make a difference. Consider the following dialogue: When you need to push the school staff on your child's behalf, remember this model and how the alternative approach might sway them toward helping and away from making your life harder.

You say: "My child has had an additional evaluation by a local expert in the area concerning his educational needs. This doctor said that the school needs to provide some additional assistance, such as one-on-one tutoring and special classroom accommodations. I know my rights."

They hear: "Do what I say or there is going to be trouble." **They think to themselves:** "Who does she think she is anyway? Her child is not the only kid in the school. We can wait her out. Besides, why should we go out of our way to help her kid?"

They say: "We are all booked up right now with testing slots. The earliest we can schedule anything will be in May. Anyway, you have to go through your classroom teacher before we can initiate anything. I am so sorry."

You say instead: "I know how backed up you are here, and I appreciate all you and all the school staff have been doing for my son. It's been just amazing. At any rate, he seems to be falling further behind, and I know you are concerned, too. I hate to put additional pressure on you at a time like this, but how can we get the testing going? Perhaps I can assist the process by getting some of the testing done in the community. It's so expensive, though. What do you suggest?"

They hear instead: "She's really pulling for her son, understandably so. We don't have any resources, unfortunately, and we're all backed up for testing. But she's been volunteering in the school. I'd sure like to help her out."

They say instead: "I'll check and see if there's any way to get him tested sooner rather than later. I'd really like to help. Don't give up on us yet!"

• *Pick your battles carefully.* How? Parents advise that if you are not sure something is worth fighting for and you feel strung out about it, you should put in on the shelf for one to two weeks. Don't even think about it, if you can avoid it. You're in this for the long run, so that amount of time won't make any difference. Then, revisit the issue. Was it worth the energy you were expending? Is it still worth it? Does your best friend agree? Do other ADHD-experienced parents agree? If not, let it go and move on. But if that is impossible—you *still* feel strongly—put it back on the shelf for another two weeks. Rarely will another two weeks hurt.

• *Anticipate problems and offer solutions.* This is an important strategy that will make it easier to create win–win solutions that others feel good about. Anticipating problems is somewhat like predicting the future, so there can be a lot of guesswork involved. But as you think and talk to others about the challenging situations you face—in school, at home, wherever—you'll get better at this over time, because history is a great teacher. Experience counts. So when facing a new situation, think about what can go wrong. Remember, you are your child's advocate. Wayne Gretzky, perhaps the greatest hockey player ever, was asked how he was so successful, and he replied, "I just skate to the place where I think the puck *is going to be.*"

Let's say you're going to an IEP meeting for your child at the beginning of the year. You don't know what to expect, but you're feeling anxious about the fact that a new teacher is scheduled to start in the middle of the year. Will she be willing to use the effective home–school behavior plan you've developed over time for your child? By thinking about what this change could bring, you've already anticipated a potential problem. You could go to the IEP meeting and demand to know how the school is going to ensure that this strategy continues to be used. But put yourself in the school staff's shoes for a minute. In doing that, all you're accomplishing is to add another burden to their load. To become effective in this situation, you need to go one step further and present some possible solutions, perhaps outlining the advantages and disadvantages of each. In this example, you might go to the IEP meeting with a handout that describes the home–school behavior plan, and request that it be included in the IEP. Or you could suggest setting up a meeting with the new teacher before she starts to discuss her experience with ADHD and see if she is more comfortable with a similar behavior plan with which she has experience; you could still make sure the IEP specifies that a home–school behavior plan agreeable to both parents and teacher be in use at all times. Now you will be helping the school staff with *their* problem, as well as resolving your own.

• *Act early and act fast.* Work early in the year with the principal to form a good relationship with her. That way, when you want to start planning for next year, you've already got a strong ally. Don't hesitate to do some detective work early in each school year. As you hook up with other parents, find out from them who the best teachers are for the next year. If you don't know this by now, you only have to experience it once to know that a given teacher, one that your child likes and thinks likes him, can make a *huge* difference in your life and that of your child—between a great year and a disastrous year. As the end of the year approaches, you want to help the principal see that the best solution for next year is to assign your child to that teacher. Notice how this is a win–win situation?

Here's the same idea in real life: "Grades 1 and 2 were a learning process and the teacher was wonderful. Between her and the guidance counselor, we worked to catch my son up with the rest of the class. We had to send him to an enrichment facility to get him caught up but, overall, the school was wonderful. Third grade was a nightmare. The teacher was a perfectionist and wouldn't settle for anything less. She would go along with the IEP plan when we were in a meeting with the principal, but she wouldn't follow it in the classroom. That year was a living nightmare. Fourth grade is much better. To avoid the problems we had in third grade, I called a meeting with both of my son's teachers, as well as the resource teacher, the speech teacher, and the principal. We went over the IEP and started the year off great. Despite fourth grade being a real challenge, it has gone well. All of the teachers, the doctors, my son, and I have worked together to come up with the best game plan. Most of all, I have tried my hardest to be supportive of everyone at school. When they know I'm on their side, it makes everything much easier."

Another story: "I start early by contacting the principal and the teacher. I let them know I want to be informed frequently of progress and problems—that I want to work with them to solve issues, that I support their expectations, and that I want processes in place to help my child succeed. I don't want my daughter to be 'beat up' and fail before we take action to help her."

And a word of advice from one parent about finding the best teacher for a child with ADHD: "I have found that the new teachers (younger) have more patience and are willing to work harder with the kids, especially the ones that are more challenging." Older teachers, in my experience, sometimes get really set in their ways, or the system wears them down. It seems to be the rare teacher who is a real veteran and retains her enthusiasm.

• *Be prepared to document your reasons for requesting a service or change for your child.* Here's what one father told me: "I have had a lot of support from our family physician regarding treatment and school supports for both our sons. I generally write a letter to the school about what I would like done, changed, and so on, and he attaches it to his letter, stating that it is his opinion that the idea should be carried out."

• *Join the PTA.* Get involved in whatever parent association or other group is available. "I am a big advocate for special ed programs," said one parent. "I joined the Committee on Special Education and attended all the meetings as a parent representative." Get to know the school board members. Remember, there is strength in numbers. If you are the only one who is causing problems for the school system, you'll have much less leverage than if you speak with and for the PTA or a group of other parents. And remember, schools tend to be quite political organizations. So the input of multiple parents is a powerful force, and keeping parents happy, particularly if it is not just a "crackpot" parent that the administrator can write off, is central to any administrator keeping his job and making the school board members happy. So find out who the other parents are whose children have similar needs. Strategize with them, and when appropriate, present your needs from the strength of a group of parents that you help organize, even if it is only three or four parents.

Parents' Top Ten: How to Be the Best School Parent You Can Be

1. "Be present as much as possible."
2. "No matter how angry you may get with particular teachers, continue to try to work as a team with them."
3. "Praise and encourage the teachers who appear to go the extra mile for your child, because if it weren't for them, your job as a parent would be a lot worse."
4. "Visit the school as much as possible. Stay involved."
5. "Above all, stay informed of your child's rights in the IEP process."
6. "Let the teachers know you are on their side, but that you always have your child's best interest at heart."
7. "Teach your children how to advocate for themselves, so that it becomes second nature to them."
8. "Never stop voicing your opinions."
9. "Keep an open and proactive relationship with the school."
10. "Be realistic about your child's situation (don't go into the school acting like your child is perfect, when you KNOW he's not. It just puts the school on the defensive and shuts down communications."

• *Volunteer to help.* Whether it's in the classroom itself, the library, or the front office, being seen and becoming known as a regular presence—a benevolent one—makes you an insider. You are part of the solution, not part of the problem; an ally, not an adversary. This strategy has the further advantage of allowing you to get a better feel for your child's problems, since you might be in a position to observe them more directly. One mother said volunteering in her child's class once a week ultimately contributed to more effective communication with the teachers, because it enabled her to get to know them better, know what goes on in class, and see the interactions with her child and others. Or if the teacher is stressed out and feels she can't take extra time for your child, giving her some of your time might relieve some stress and make her more able and willing to assist your child. Other means of helping might be working on the school fund-raisers, or helping secure additional resources such as furniture, computers, and so forth. "I always signed up for field trips so I knew the teacher wouldn't have to deal with the impulsive behaviors out in the community," said one mom.

Making Your Child's Teacher(s) Work for You

Having your child's teacher in his or her corner will pay huge dividends throughout the school year. But the teacher may have as many as thirty sets of parents, not just one. That's a lot of corners. What is a reasonable expectation and what is not?

What You Should Expect from Your Child's Teacher

Respond to Your Requests for Information about Your Child's Progress

As you know, regular times are set up throughout the school year for teachers to give parents feedback—in most schools anywhere from two to four conferences, more for younger children, and fewer as they get older. But those parent–teacher meetings are set up to serve as a *minimum* level of communication between the two of you. Your child has special needs, greater than many of the other children in the classroom, so close coordination is essential. You want to be able to give your child positive feedback for giving his best effort at school, and the only way to give that feedback soon enough for it to count is probably to confer with the teacher weekly, more often in crisis situations, less often, perhaps only monthly, when things are stable. "Be involved with the child's school," advised one parent. "Let the teachers know you are concerned with what goes on in the life of your child. Call regular conferences just to discuss how things are going, if there is something you need to know about."

For elementary school children, you may be able to set up a routine for this communication, using something like the "daily report card" (DRC), a convenient tool that allows efficient communication between home and school. Using the DRC, simply a single sheet of paper with ratings of the child's performance for each of the items that day, along with the teacher's initials, the parent, teacher, and child work on an agreed-on, small (four to five) set of target behaviors for the child. The child's task is to bring home the DRC every day. The teacher's job is to fill it out (thirty seconds to one minute). Your task is to encourage your child when she is struggling, and to praise and reward her when she succeeds. You'll also need to take time to set up a reward system with your child (see Appendix I).

Ensure That You Know about Your Child's Homework Assignments

Along with the DRC, you may want to include a place for the teacher to note your child's homework assignments. Or assignments might be written down by the child in a little notebook and initialed by the teacher. This way, the teacher does not have to write down each assignment for each child (increasingly hard to do as the number of children with special needs mounts). Instead, your child has this responsibility, along with the task of getting the teacher's signature or initials on what he has written down. Everyone is in the loop. As children get older, or as tasks get more complex, some teachers will give out a homework sheet, where task assignments, particularly longer term projects, are spelled out more clearly. You might suggest this, but be sure to ask whether this strategy seems like it might work for your child's teacher and whether the assignments lend themselves to it. Otherwise, from the teacher's perspective, you may be recommending more work for him. Is there anything you could do to help here?

Be Concerned

Your child's teacher should show genuine concern and care about your child and her progress. He should make your child feel welcome and liked in the classroom. How can you tell if this is the case? In many instances, the child will like the teacher because she feels valued and liked in return. So if your child doesn't feel that way, it could mean that the teacher, however well intentioned, may not be communicating it effectively or in a way your child can appreciate it. You might help by juicing the system a little. If you are convinced it is true, tell your child that Mr. So-and-So *does* like her. Give your child a little gift that she can give to the teacher to add a bit more life to their interactions. If you think the teacher can hear and respond well to the information, share your concerns with him. Sometimes teachers are busy and may not realize that a child feels that way. Drawing it to their attention may help them go out of their way to communicate their caring for your child.

But sometimes you feel that the teacher actually *does not* like your child. This is a problem. If you feel it, your child probably does as well. Here, you may have to try a number of strategies to see if you can change things around. The "apple for the teacher" trick might help. Your working to form a good relationship with the teacher is another useful approach. Is she actually this way with all children? If so, this could be tougher to turn around.

Avoid Punitive Approaches with Your Child

"Almost the first day in kindergarten," remembered one mother, "the teacher said she could not conduct a reading class, that she had to squeeze our child between her knees as she sat in the chair; he would pull other children's hair, bite them, and so on. Schools at times have been more punitive than understanding of the condition, are often short-staffed and underfunded, and therefore cannot zero in on handling these special situations." This is worrisome. In this situation, the teacher may not only communicate active dislike, but she may also actually use approaches that set your child's jaw or make him want to avoid the class. Unduly or frequently restricting recess, berating your child, drawing negative attention to him in front of the class, and assigning tedious make-work tasks intended to punish are all no-nos, certainly if they become a pattern. Yes, your child may have behavioral difficulties, and no, you do not want to make excuses for your child. But there are effective strategies for dealing with these problems, and punitive approaches coupled with a poor teacher–child relationship make an explosive combination.

Make Any Necessary (Though Modest) Classroom Accommodations

Accommodations should be aimed at counteracting your child's difficulties to make the child's school day work out better. These can include seating arrangements, homework accommodations, a system to inform you of the day's assignments, and similar measures. If you get the impression that your child's teachers and other school staff may not be familiar with the techniques that work best with children who have ADHD, suggestions that you can offer are listed on page 159 under "Tips for Parents to Share with Teachers." Remember, these should be posed as *suggestions*, not demands. You want to leave the teacher wanting to work with you. Also, keep in mind that not all techniques will work with every child, so you should look for opportunities to help the teacher find appropriate modifications and accommodations that help maximize your child's potential and productivity, based on your knowledge of your child.

Put In at Least a Little Extra Time

Yes, it does take a bit of extra time. But again, the laws require that such accommodations be made for children with disabilities. You can often find strategies to keep the teacher's additional time investment to a minimum, such as using the DRC or having your child write the homework assignments down, with the teacher needing only to initial the page. Regardless, the time and effort needed to provide your child with necessary accommodations shouldn't mean that your child gets shorted on other needs. And, remember, when you're asking a teacher to put in a *little* extra time, you're not asking for the moon. After all, some teachers take it upon themselves to go the extra mile every day: "We were lucky that our child had a phenomenal special ed teacher who has worked with her for the last three years to get her into a mainstream classroom."

Taking Charge: How to Get What You Need from Your Child's Teacher

Working with a child with ADHD can place a burden on teachers. But you probably already know that a good teacher can make a tremendous difference in your child's (and your) life. The most effective teacher for children with ADHD uses a mix of patience, structure, positive discipline, consistency, and nurturance. Effective teachers of children with ADHD keep the children engaged in learning by using a varied, multisensory teaching style, getting responses from them, calling their names during instruction, and using exciting examples and illustrations, and frequent praise for attention and correct responses.

How hard it is to get this kind of teaching for your child will depend on what you and the teacher are up against. If the student–teacher ratio in your child's school is low, the teachers are fairly knowledgeable about ADHD, and they seem genuinely dedicated to giving all their students an equal opportunity to learn, you're way ahead of the game. The only other ingredient you may need to optimize your child's school experience is a productive partnership with the teachers. A good partnership is even more critical when teachers have too many students, too little knowledge of ADHD, and are simply worn out by all the demands placed on them, including those from other parents. Regardless of the circumstances at the school, the education of children is a responsibility that must be *shared* by the teacher and parent as *partners*. Teachers need to recognize what a powerful asset a parent can be; parents need to appreciate what a powerful component teachers are to a child's success.

Partnering with Your Child's Teacher(s)

As a parent, you can expect and receive cooperation from most teachers by appreciating and relying on their expertise, recognizing the difficulties inherent in their job, and informing them about what your child needs and responds well to. As one wise mother said, "Be on the lookout for teachers and individuals who don't understand ADHD. Don't let them become your enemy. It is very difficult to get their help if they think you are an enemy. Instead, form a team and work as a team toward a common goal for the betterment of your child." Remember how crucial you are to that team. As one parent described it,

> "Teachers mean well, but don't take them too seriously with regard to the severity of your child's behavior or symptoms. Kids with ADHD need a little help sometimes. Teachers who have not taken the time to recognize your child's triggers or cues may jump to extreme conclusions. As parents, we learn little tricks to avoid some of the typical ADHD problems. Teachers may not realize that your child may simply need a few reminders to do a task, or a little verbal encouragement to finish that worksheet."

You need to approach teachers and school personnel in an open, nondefensive, yet assertive way. Think of each one as an individual who really wants to do the best job possible, despite often being overwhelmed. This is usually correct and always the best way to approach them. As a result, we must also show our appreciation to the teacher and the school when they do something well. Positive changes in student achievement, attitude, and behavior can occur when teachers and parents are partners in promoting the learning and success of a child with ADHD.

Making the Partnership Work

In every interaction with the child's teacher, you can be actively building an effective partnership. To make that partnership work you should do the following:

• Communicate your concern from the beginning of the school year. One parent described how she would sit down with her child's teachers to talk about her son's ADHD and the strategies that had been effective for him in school in the past, from putting him up front in the classroom to assigning him special jobs. The latter had a double benefit: Keeping him busy eliminated a lot of opportunities to "fail" at sitting still, and giving him a unique task made him feel different in a positive way instead of constantly in a negative way.

• Establish positive, frequent communication. Drop the teacher a note telling him how much you appreciate him when you see any positive effort on his part. Make sure he knows you, likes you, and wants to go out of his way for you.

• Ask parents whose children had this teacher last year what kinds of approaches worked best with him.

• Consider using a DRC to communicate success, concerns, or skills to work on (see page 154).

• Take every opportunity to show that you appreciate the teacher. For example, find out her birthday and have your child bring a small gift to class. Bring in a cake on that day and lead the kids in singing "Happy Birthday." Or bake cookies for her and the class on Valentine's Day.

• Keep the teacher informed of any important changes in your child's life or treatment. If you have found some technique that seems to work particularly well, share it with him. He may want to apply it as well. Or if your child is upset and bothered about something, let the teacher know, so he can anticipate any new behavior or mood problems and respond in a helpful manner.

• Talk to the teacher at the first sign of a problem.

• Coordinate a behavior management program with the teacher, so everyone is working on the same thing. But what if the teacher already feels beleaguered and views your proposing the program you're using at home as just another big chore? You might offer ways for the teacher to put better programs into place. So if the teacher doesn't have a star chart or school–home reward system in place, you might give her the actual materials needed. Ask what behaviors she would like you to encourage your child to exhibit in class by using rewards at home. Then find ways to work together to modify the materials for your child's and the classroom's needs, based on the teacher's input.

• Make school behavior and academic success part of your child's reward program at home, such as by using the DRC.

• How about asking the teacher what you could do to make her life easier? Maybe offer to volunteer in some way that has nothing to do with your own child (maybe the teacher really needs help with coaching kids in the classroom in their writing projects, and that might free her up to do something that you'll want for your own child later).

• Ask the teacher whether there are other parents dealing with the same problems, and whether they'd be willing to talk to you so that you could share strategies that each has discovered help the kids' classroom behavior. This might also make the teacher's classroom run better. What's not to like about this?

• Ask the teacher if she needs any supplies for the classroom. We hear more and more about how teachers spend their own money on supplies or depend on donations from parents—for things large and small.

As partnerships grow, trust also grows, and it may be appropriate and useful for you to share information with the teacher, not only about your child but also about larger issues in ADHD. As you get more expert, it is very likely that you may know more about ADHD than the teacher, and what kinds of classroom strategies work and don't work for your child. So here are a few tips you can share. Remember, teachers don't particularly want you to tell them their business, so tact and timing are key. It might work for you to give teachers the tips as a handout, or you might find a chance to subtly share them on an as-needed basis, even if only one at a time.

Tips for Parents to Share with Teachers

• Provide the student with structured and predictable learning spaces.
  —Post daily rules, schedules, and assignments.
  —Call attention to schedule changes.
  —Set specific times for specific tasks.
  —Plan academic subjects for the morning hours.
  —Design a quiet work space for use upon request.
  —Seat the child with a positive peer model.
  —Provide regularly scheduled and frequent breaks.
  —Use attention-getting devices (e.g., secret signals, color codes, etc.).

• Modify the curriculum.
  —Mix high- and low-interest activities.
  —Provide computerized learning materials.
  —Simplify and increase visual presentation.
  —Use visual reference for auditory instruction.
  —Teach organization and study skills.
  —Use learning strategies such as mnemonic devices and links.

• Channel excessive activity into acceptable avenues; use activity as a reward and active responses in instruction.
  —Encourage directed movement in the classroom or allow standing during seatwork.
  —Reward appropriate behavior by allowing the child to run an errand or clean the board.
  —Use activities that encourage talking, moving, organizing, or working at the board.

- Offer substitute verbal or motor responses to make while the child is waiting, or allow daydreaming or planning during this time.
  —Teach the child to continue on easier parts of the task, or doodle or play with clay to fill up time while waiting.
  —Direct impatience or bossiness into leadership (e.g., paper passer, line reader).

- Decrease the length of the task or make tasks more interesting to help sustain attention during routine tasks and activities.
  —Break one task into smaller parts, or give fewer spelling words or math problems.
  —Allow students to work with partners or make a game out of checking work.

- Increase the choice and specific interest of tasks for the student to encourage compliance and completion of tasks.
  —Provide a limited choice of tasks, topics, and activities, and use preferred activities as incentives.
  —Fit tasks with the student's learning abilities and preferred response style by offering various ways to respond and various degrees of difficulty.

- Ease the difficulty of beginning a new task by providing structure and highlighting important parts.
  —Encourage note taking and provide written directions, as well as oral ones, and state the standards of acceptable work.

- Help the child complete assignments on time by increasing the use of lists and assignment organizers.
  —Establish routines for handing in and retrieving assignments and encourage the student to ask the question "Do I have everything?" when leaving one place for another.

EXERCISE 3

Role Playing the Parent–Teacher Partnership

Try the following exercises to practice communicating and collaborating with your child's teacher.

Role Play 1

Work with another parent and role-play that one of you is a concerned parent and the other is the child's teacher.

Teacher: As the teacher, you should take on the role of a concerned teacher, who is ready and willing to cooperate with the parent. The teacher is asked by the parent to meet with him to talk about concerns the parent has with his child.

Parent: Your child has recently received a diagnosis of ADHD. You want to talk with your child's teacher about what she should know about ADHD and how this disorder may affect your child in the classroom or other areas at school.

- Practice explaining your child's diagnosis to the teacher using language learned throughout this book. Using the "Tips for Parents to Share with Teachers," practice suggesting specific tips the teacher could use in the classroom that may work well with your child.
- Remember that these tips should not be communicated as demands or expectations placed on the teacher. Instead, offer them as helpful suggestions that will make the classroom environment better for the child and the teacher's job easier.
- Work together with the teacher through open dialogue to discuss what may or may not work best with the child in the classroom, and discuss any modifications to the given techniques deemed appropriate. Illustrate these changes by writing them down on paper and coming up with examples of when problems may occur and how to work through them.

Role Play 2

Using the same circumstances, this time the person acting as the teacher adopts a resistant attitude, so the parent can practice communicating with a teacher who may not be as open to suggestions for what to do in the classroom.

Teacher: As the teacher, you should act as difficult as possible in communicating with the parent about her child's diagnosis. You do not want to change the way you teach in the classroom in any way, especially for one child. You are also uneasy about how this type of disorder will affect other students and what it will mean in terms of extra work for you.

Parent: As the parent, you are now trying to work with a teacher who does not really want to work with you. Practice being assertive without being aggressive. Make sure the teacher knows that you are there not only out of concern for your child but also to help the teacher develop new ways of communicating with the child in the classroom, making his job and relationship with the child a more positive experience. Be sure to explain simply and clearly what an ADHD diagnosis means and, being sure to *work with the teacher,* walk though ways in which the teacher can modify teaching strategies in the classroom.

Switch roles and repeat each exercise!

Terrific Tips from Parents: Working Effectively with Teachers

- "I keep insisting on regular exercise during the school day and tell the school that if he could help it he would, that it is a recognized disorder, he has been diagnosed severely hyperactive. I relate that my child keeps saying he has this 'bundle of energy' he needs to release; I feel these children can be mainstreamed but need an extra teacher/assistant to work intensively with these 'intense' children! I repeatedly tell them that this is a result of his ADHD, making sure each teacher knows this."

• "I found that our cooperation and working with rather than against teachers was conducive to getting Michael these minimal yet essential adaptations. Seating him toward the front of the room away from windows was a very simple measure that diminished sources of distraction for him. Having timed tests with a silent rather than a ticking timer made a big difference for him. We found an assignment book at a teachers' supply store that had a special daily area for 'Things to Remember,' 'Things to Take to/from School,' and 'Long-Term Assignments,' in addition to the normal subject list."

What to Do When Things Go Wrong

So what do you do when your child's teacher seems increasingly intolerant of your child's difficulties and wants to respond punitively (such as with suspension or other disciplinary actions)? How about if teachers or staff don't want to apply appropriate accommodations? What should you do when the teacher seems hostile to you or skeptical that your child has a disability? How about if your child says he doesn't like the teacher or that the teacher is "mean"? Or if the teacher doesn't return your phone calls or puts you off when you request a meeting, or expects too little from your child? Under such conditions, you may find it difficult to establish a good partnership with your child's teacher. In the event of a difficult relationship, it is important to continue working toward a partnership for the benefit of your child. Try the following:

- Address the teacher directly with your concerns.
- Provide the teacher with information on ADHD.
- Call a school support team or an IEP meeting if your child has an IEP.
- Speak candidly and confidentially to the principal, asking for advice on how to deal with the teacher.
- Find out from other parents (in this year or past years) what they may have tried to do that seemed to work with this teacher.
- Find ways to agree with the teacher and build on those points of agreement.
- Avoid saying "You should . . ."; instead, say "I wonder if we did. . . ."
- Find out if the parents of your child's classmates have similar concerns and, if so, what good strategies they have used with this teacher. Band together to approach the teacher and, if necessary, present your concerns about this teacher to the principal.

EXERCISE 4

How to Get a Teacher Who Is "Just Too Busy" to Work with You on a Home–School Reward System

Read the following dialogue, then practice saying your part in the mirror. Remember, don't blink, don't hesitate.

YOU: I learned from the doctor that there is a special program we can use to help Joey stay on track during class time. It involves a special reward program for Joey, based on regular feedback between you and me, using what the doctor calls a "daily report card." Have you heard of this? What do you think?

TEACHER: I really don't have time to spend in any one-on-one situation with a single child. It's important for children to learn to take responsibility for themselves. Besides, I have too much work to do to take time for this.

YOU: I know how busy you must be. I don't know how you get it all done. So I am wondering, what can we do that will really keep the burden on you very low, yet still allow Joey to do his very best?

TEACHER: It is important for Joey to learn responsibility, and at this age (nine), he should be doing it by himself.

YOU: I know this is a lot to ask of you, but we need to find a way to motivate him to do his best in your classroom. How about if I bring in the materials the doctor gave me for a home–school reward program, and we go over it? It'll only take a few minutes of your time, and I think it will save you a lot of time with Joey over the long run. Would it help if I brought you the doctor's note?

TEACHER: OK, let's try it, but just for the next few weeks.

Or if she says: "It is a lot to ask, and I just can't do this for every child!"

You wait a week or two, send her a nice note apologizing for catching her at a bad time, and offer to help her in her class. Or try again. She probably felt bad about her response. If she responds similarly, after further attempts at reconciliation on your part, hang on. Either stick it out, get some more advice from other parents who have worked with her before, speak to the principal, or request a change if things have gotten really tense.

School Peer-Relationship Problems

Throughout this chapter, we've been concentrating on getting the most out of the schools so your child can succeed academically. But we all know that school is usually a child's most significant social arena, too, if for no other reason than that kids spend most of their day there. Remember that it's critical to their self-esteem that they succeed in the social parts of school, too. For many kids, extracurricular activities provide a structured social milieu as well as an opportunity to be good at something besides academics. See Chapter 8 for tips on maximizing these opportunities. However, for school settings, consider the following points from parents:

"I did a research project for CHADD a few years back on school discipline. I have over 700 stories of how kids were bullied in the schools and the schools most often punished the child with ADHD for lashing out at the bullies. (The connection between this and ADHD is that youth with ADHD are often the targets of bullying behavior—described as 'provocative victims' by Dan Olweus, founder of the Bullying Prevention Program that I am now training schools on.)"

Or as another parent reported,

"My son's 504 plan is in place and seems to be working; he likes his teacher, his grades are going up, but he still tries to skip school, and we've recently found out that it's because he's still being bullied and harassed at school. He's one of the so-called 'provocative victims,' and he's had problems long enough that it's almost impossible for him to change his image at school. How can we address this critical problem when we seem to have used up all of the school administration and faculty's goodwill just getting special ed assistance?"

So what do you do when . . .

• *A kid comes home upset because he's constantly teased, yet the teacher supposedly does nothing about it?* Tough question, with too few good answers. The best long-term solution that will help everybody is to get the school to learn about and introduce the Olweus programs into the school. There are among the best-studied programs shown to reduce bullying and playground violence in the world, and if implemented, they get the whole school (including the teacher who always looks the other way) to recognize and systematically address these problems. But that is a long-term plan. In the meantime, you might raise the issue with the principal, asking to speak with him "in confidence" if it seems appropriate (you don't want him or the teacher saying something back to your child), and asking for his input on what he thinks is going on. Remember, you have only your child's version of the story. If the complete story suggests that the teacher is ignoring bullying, you might ask for the principal's assistance in addressing the problem and offer to help in any way you can. Principals are pretty sensitive to this stuff, since school systems often feel liable if they know about a problem and do nothing to address it. Follow up your conversation with a thank-you note. If the problem continues, speak to the principal again, and again offer your assistance. See if other parents share your concern (some certainly do), and make it an issue for the PTA to raise as a concern.

• *You get calls from parents saying your child is bullying the other kids at recess?* This happens too, of course. Is your child being fully and appropriately treated? Do you have a behavior plan in place to address the problem? Bullying is an excellent and quite responsive target for behavior therapies, but it may require a professional's assistance. Don't go it alone if things are not working. Also explore whether your child's medication, if any, is adjusted adequately. Many aggressive and oppositional symptoms respond to the traditional ADHD treatments, such as the stimulants.

Your Action Plan

Remember your action plan created in Chapter 3? Pull it out. You need to figure out how to fit these folks into the plan. It might be a good idea to share the plan with your child's teacher and special education staff. Discuss the special needs your child has and show them what you are doing to meet the child's needs. Point out where the school can be of special assistance in this plan, and ask explicitly where they think they can contribute. Don't take no for an answer, and remember to use the broken record technique if your initial requests seem to fall on deaf ears: "I know how busy you are, but I really need some additional help on this for Johnny to succeed, which, of course, is what we all want. And I know you want to meet all of the special education and IDEA requirements. So what do you think would be the best way for the school to increase its involvement and assistance?" (Repeat as often as needed!)

Before leaving this chapter, refer to your short- and intermediate-term action plans. Are there additional areas that need to be filled in? Have you spotted any additional educational needs, approaches that can be taken, or ultimate objectives? See some of the examples I have entered into the Intermediate-Term Action Plan on the next page, then do your own (see the blank in Appendix F).

"After fighting for five years to get help for my son in school, in fifth grade, his teacher said to me at our first conference, 'I think Terrence has a learning disability.' Finally, someone validated what I had been feeling and believed for all those years. She was our angel. When all else seemed hopeless, I prayed."

"Through the years, our experience with the school system has been all over the map, from extremely positive to highly negative. There is a definite need for more education about the societal impact and the educator's role in this disorder."

"Your child's ability to succeed will be a lot better with medication assistance, if it is doctor-recommended. I can assure you that your child will make his own decision in time as to whether he wants to continue his medication (usually around middle school). Get an IEP in place as soon as possible to protect his rights and accommodate for special needs."

"Fortunately, I have never had any problems with my child's schools. He has been in four schools since he was diagnosed, and we have been blessed with wonderful teachers. I go in at the beginning of the school year and talk to all his teachers, informing them that he has ADHD. I say that I am happy to answer any questions that they may have. I also let them know what they can expect out of him, from me as his parent, and that if they see any problem that needs to be addressed, I am ALWAYS available for them. I think that the key to success in your child's school is to be as involved as possible. The teachers need to know that you are concerned and that you are willing to make yourself available for any conferences. I also call regular conferences with his teachers, and we discuss how things are going and what he needs to work on."

INTERMEDIATE-TERM ACTION PLAN

Your child's needs	Approaches How will the need(s) be addressed? Resources?	Who will do it? Who else will assist and be on your child's team?	When? What is the time frame for accomplishing specific tasks?	Outcomes Intermediate-term goals and objectives
Social–emotional needs				
Medical needs	Get doctor's letter to request IEP and special ed services for reading	Me	Call for appointment	Strong medical support for IEP!
Educational needs 1. Needs to improve reading—behind grade	Get outside testing done to document that he is behind two grades, then get IEP scheduled	Use my friend's recommendation for a psychologist	Testing to be done in next two months (Nov.). IEP by Jan. School services to begin ASAP. Hire tutor if IEP stalls	Move up one reading level, from third to fourth grade, by end of next summer
2. Expand his talents in math so he can feel he is "really good at it"	Enroll him for math camp this summer	Husband to check with coworker with a math-whiz son on best camp recommendation		
Parent–family needs				

166

Seven

GETTING THE BEST OUT OF YOUR HOME AND FAMILY LIFE

"We need to be careful not to compare our children or our families with others. Wishin' and hopin' devalues the child that you have and makes it impossible for him to succeed."

"Some days, by the end of the day, I am so exhausted. I just want her to go away so I can have some time to myself."

"Until the testing and diagnosis, even my husband felt our son must be just lazy and unmotivated and acting out. This had a significant impact on the relationship between my husband and my son."

Schools may come and go, and you may end up switching doctors, therapists, or healthcare plans. Families and family members, however, cannot be replaced. You are in this family for the long run, and if you all are going to come out of this alive, the trick is learning how make this family work for you and for the other members as well. Our families have many functions, from supplying our physical needs to filling our emotional needs, to managing the ins and outs of daily life. This chapter covers that entire range, from handling the daily routines, to making relationships more satisfactory, to filling your own personal needs for support, time alone, and intermittent relief from the constant demands placed on you as a parent of a child with ADHD.

Making Your Relationship with Your Child Work for You

"It was the most painful experience of my life . . . feeling like my own child hated me, resented me. And I felt so guilty when I realized I didn't want to be around him. I knew I loved him as his mother, but I felt like I hated him. That's so hard to think and say, and embarrassing to admit. But I now know lots of others have been through this too."

Throughout this book, we've been talking about getting things done for your child if your son or daughter with ADHD is simply the passive recipient of all your achievements. In fact, of course, the child plays a big role in how well you collectively manage his disorder. How he behaves at home—whether the issue is chores, sibling relationships, parent–child bonding, or homework or family activities—will determine not only how well he does in life but also how well the entire family functions as a unit. We'll talk about household routines and other practical matters later in this chapter, but first, let's look at how you view your child overall, what you expect from him, and how he fits into the family scheme.

What to Expect from Your Child with ADHD

Understanding without Excuses

How do you strike the balance between accepting the fact that your child has a behavioral condition—even a disability—and teaching the very same child to be responsible for his or her behavior? That is one of the great paradoxes that parents who have a child with ADHD must learn to grapple with and fully integrate into their parenting, their loving, and their disciplining of this child. This is the cornerstone of your success, the most important and difficult thing that you will have to master as a truly expert parent. Yet this is what I learned—the hard way, through tears, anger, and anguish. And this is what so many of the parents learned who have given us the gifts of their poignant personal stories: Parents constantly brought up the fact that you have to love and accept your child, but that that doesn't mean making excuses.

Remember principle 13 from Chapter 2? *Acceptance*. In the deepest way, this attitude—ironically, for many parents, even an *attitude of gratitude*—stands as their greatest achievement en route to becoming an expert parent of a youngster with ADHD. This attitude combines an unfailing love for one's offspring with the setting of appropriate standards of behavior and achievement, just as you do with and for your other kids. Parents' own words say it best: "And always remember . . . the child can no more help having ADHD than diabetes or cancer. He cannot 'snap' out of it. Understand his limitations, but help him find areas where he can excel. Help him understand his limitations without allowing him to use his disability as an excuse. It's a very fine line. But defining it and walking it is a must." This takes constant vigilance as a parent, so that you deal with your own personal feelings toward your child, not just your child's behavior: "Your ADHD child is not broken. She is just wired differently. Love her for who she is, not what you thought she would be. The future is as bright for her as it is for children without ADHD."

These children must learn to love and accept themselves, a harder task even than that of the parents: "Remember that ADHD children can be sensitive and are limited at times with what they can achieve. Do not communicate that you are disappointed in who they are. Rather, teach them to accept themselves and arm them with knowledge." Or as another parent put it, "Just love your child. Take numerous deep breaths a day and remember it's *not* their fault (or yours). Helping them to find ways to succeed will be key."

They are really going to need your help if they are to do this. And remember, they will have to endure the confusing, sometimes paralyzing transitions between acceptance and encouragement at home, and rejection and discouragement everywhere else. Yet how else can we as parents help them counteract the loss of self-esteem that occurs because of all these losses of personal relationships in the challenging outside world, on top of the temporary setbacks that such children (and their parents) inevitably experience at home?

> "The transitions are difficult for me (to rehash our life history again and again) and for my son to lose a 'friend' and re-bond with a stranger. He felt a great deal of loss in being repeatedly tossed from day care programs; he never understood why they didn't like him anymore. Then you have a physician or therapist move you on to another doc, and it starts all over again. It is very difficult to maintain the child's self-esteem when he gets passed from place to place."

As this parent knows without actually saying it, this attitude of acceptance and understanding—without excuses—is the very hallmark of her love for her child, a love remarkable for its resilience and endurance despite all she has had to go through as a parent. If only we could see and feel this from the very beginning with these kids!

Uncertainty and Unpredictability

But life is uncertain and always more complicated and so much messier than it seems from a 35,000-foot altitude. So while we're putting all this effort into trying to make things better, we're still going to have to live with the idea of expecting the unexpected from our child. Impulsivity means that, as parents, we can't necessarily predict what these kids will do any more than our kids themselves can—what they do doesn't fit normal patterns of behavior, does it?

> "The most difficult thing for me is not knowing what to expect from my son and his behavior. Harold is our first child, and in the beginning, my husband and I thought that all two-and-a-half-year-olds acted as 'busy' as he did. But then I'd see him playing with other children his age, and his learning was definitely behind. He couldn't focus on toys like the other kids. His mind seemed to ricochet from one activity to the next, and his body had difficulty keeping up. It was like a slap in the face that we needed help. But even now, with doctors, therapy, and medication, it is very difficult to know what to expect from him and how to set up boundaries."

Ironically, when we reach "the right place" inside ourselves as parents, the unpredictability is sometimes one of the more lovable, but still problematic, aspects of these kids' behavior.

> "Prior to my son's being diagnosed with ADHD, he played soccer. In one game, he was on the field, and the ball was hit to him. Well, at the same time, the wind had picked up and was filling his shirt. Needless to say, he was *so* entranced by this he failed to notice the ball at his feet and the twenty to thirty people screaming on the sidelines, 'Kick the ball!' His game improved dramatically after medication."

Taking Charge of Your Relationship with Your Child

Be Honest with Your Child about His or Her Condition

Personally, I am convinced that if you hide the disorder from the child, he may in fact think he's "bad," and his self-esteem will plummet. And in another cruel twist of fate, if you blame yourself for the problem, the child inevitably, and without even knowing, will take advantage of it:

> "I have *huge* issues with parents who don't tell their child with ADHD that he has it. I think the one thing that really needs to be attended to is your honesty with your child and accepting of it. You are your child's best advocate, and if you don't believe in it or trust it, then the outcomes for the child may not be as beneficial as they could be."

Furthermore, when you talk with your child about ADHD, it need not and should not be all "bad":

> "Tell your child over and over how special he is and that you love him no matter what. *And* there is a silver lining—that while he is challenging, he is also gifted with great energy and enthusiasm (which our son is!)." Or as another wise parent stated, "Love your child. They can be so much fun, and they, too, find it frustrating dealing with their ADHD."

But Am I Normal?

Yet another paradox is the fact that these kids have to feel normal even though they are "special." One parent captured this beautifully:

> "We've always been very open with our son about ADHD and what it is and how it affects him. What made him accept his 'disorder' without question was knowing that other people, especially people he knows well and can relate to, also have ADHD. So we were talking one night at bedtime, and he was feeling a little bit isolated and lonely and said that he thought ADHD made him *different* from everyone else. I tried to explain to him that everyone is different in one way or another, either by looks, or ability, or ADHD, or something else, but inside we all have a heart that loves and sustains us. He didn't get it. So I said, 'Did you know that a lot of other people have ADHD?' That caught his attention a bit, so I continued. 'Did you know that Grandpa has it?' He adores his grandpa, so he really began to listen. I said, 'Your cousin Carl [his favorite family idol] has it; so do Tommy and Michael and David [his friends]. Did you know that?' He turned to me and said, 'Mom, but they're not *different*,' and I said, 'You're absolutely right . . . ADHD isn't a bad thing; it just helps to make them who they are, just like it helps you be you . . . and we wouldn't want you any other way!' He turned to me and gave me a huge smile and hug. At that point he knew it was OK."

These children need "heroes" that give them ideas about how they too might become successful adults, as this parent points out:

> "Following dinner after an appointment at Mass General, we bumped into Ned Hallowell and his family dining next to us. I had his book in the car, and he signed it for me. He told my daughter, 'Your mind is a race car, a fabulous race car with many great ideas. . . . Grasp onto one and hold on. . . . You are truly special,' and he is a wonderful person; Tamara was so proud that she had met him. It impacted her that he was an author—he had the same disability as her, and look what he had accomplished!"

One More Time: Don't Indulge in Self-Blame

Remember, blaming yourself and wallowing in feelings of guilt may inadvertently plant in your child negative views of himself: He may feel guilty that his behavior has made you feel bad. Or if he finds guilt an especially painful feeling to bear, it may be easier for him to be angry with you for *your* emotions and distance himself from you. At least this way he won't have to feel he's to blame, because somehow it's your fault! This sets up an unstable situation that can easily lead to a child manipulating a parent. And to cap it off, the same self-blame may prevent you from being firm when needed, yet simultaneously supportive and understanding.

As you can see, guilt and self-blame are very destructive emotions, whether in you or your child. Much more helpful and productive is a problem-solving attitude: candidly and openly admitting and accepting that you have made a mistake; apologizing, if appropriate, or fixing what can be fixed, and then moving on. You want to model this and encourage the same in your child. Don't sweat it; it is hard for all of us as parents not to feel guilty for one thing or another about our children, especially about these children!

Guilt comes in many forms, so look out for the various ways we find to apply it to ourselves: "After my son's diagnosis, I was diagnosed as well with ADD (without the hyperactivity). I think I still hold misplaced guilt that it was somehow my 'fault' that he has all these problems, and that I didn't give my husband the child he'd expected. I am working through these issues. Counseling (group and individual) has been my greatest source of information in dealing with his ADHD. The public's misconceptions have been a major thorn as have been my own misconceptions."

This parent seems to have gotten a good handle on the issues and is much more likely to find ways to be able to walk that fine line of understanding without excuses, helping her children deal with their misbehaviors and infractions, learn from them, and move on.

Use Punishment Judiciously, Rewards Generously

As you have found out (you probably wouldn't be reading this book otherwise), there are all kinds of methods that work and don't work for children with ADHD. Most of us get very experienced in things that don't work, which includes even good old-fashioned parenting. What works for most kids usually does not work for kids with ADHD. And some things that you can get away with in the case of most kids may even blow up with these kids, as this parent points out: "Yelling or spanking does not work with kids with ADHD! It could even make the behavior worse. When I yell, my son will yell louder. Spanking just gives my son more drive to his disproportionate attitude. It seems to escalate his internal drive to conquer the battle, his win-at-any-cost mentality. Sad to say, but my son is only six." For these kids, behavior therapy, taught to and applied by the parents, is a much better way to go.

Use Behavior Therapy for Your Child

Behavior therapy is basically a very carefully thought through, structured, re-searched, and delivered means of giving your child rewards and punishments. If you haven't used them already, these strategies are invaluable, and you need to make them part of your regular arsenal. The best of these programs rely first on establishing/ensuring a positive relationship between parent and child. Why? A child who resents you and thinks you are unfair will think your behavior program is unfair as well and will fight it every step of the way.

Next, parent-delivered behavior therapy is structured so that parents first use the mildest procedures possible that will shape or redirect the child's behavior, such as establishing house rules (if not already in place), praising appropriate behavior, and ignoring low-level inappropriate behaviors. Of note, use of the mildest proce-dures alone (e.g., praise and ignore) is usually *not* sufficient, and some type of nega-tive "consequences" or punishment (time-out, loss of privileges, loss of points in a behavior point program) is usually necessary. Parents also learn how to give effective commands, how to develop daily charts and reward systems to encourage positive behavior and discourage negative behavior, and how to use time-out effectively.

One nice thing is that behavior programs can be applied to kids of all ages, from very young children to adolescents, even though various adaptations are needed to take age issues into account: One parent advises, "For little ones, prior to diagnosis, I strongly recommend the 1-2-3 Magic strategy. It worked very well for my child with ADHD." With adolescents, variations in procedures are needed, because adoles-cents' role in self-direction is critical. As a result, behavior systems for them usually involve contracting/negotiating with them, while still using some type of reward and consequence system.

In my experience, a star chart, point system, or some other type of daily rewards and consequences program is a must, and you will need to use them in one form or another for much of your child's growing-up years. They not only are effective behavior management tools, but they can also help you keep your temper and frus-tration at a low level. Why? Because if you put a behavior program into place, you don't have to get upset: You have a chart system with its own rewards and conse-quences, and it will be effective all by itself—in fact, more effective when you *don't* get upset.

There is no foolproof approach, and as parents we have to stay on our toes:

"One thing I learned with my child is that no discipline strategy lasts for long—you have to be creative." Another parent cautioned,

> "I had always had structures in place for my children, such as a set bedtime routine, homework time, limited TV viewing. The therapist was happy to know this and suggested only very limited behavior modification plans. He offered no help when one child (at the age of six) ripped the chart down and said that she was just not going to do it. Of course, I felt like a bad parent when the therapist told me I must be doing something wrong, since my description of the child was not what he was seeing during their sessions. He could not explain why the behavior modification was working well with my other child with ADHD. I finally found a different therapist for my six-year-old, who is now 17."

The problem this second parent encountered was likely not so much that the behavior therapy "didn't work," but that the therapist did not know how to debug the problem this parent encountered.

You will have to experiment with what rewards and consequences will work for your child. Every child is different, and what works today may not work next month with the same child. Open discussion and communication in a straightforward, nonangry way will facilitate your finding the right approach for your child, even getting her input:

> "I put my son in time-out for mouthing back to me. While in time-out, he punched a hole in the wall (this was an eight-year-old). It was later in the day when his meds had worn off—he was mad and he demonstrated lack of self-control/impulsive behavior. I had taught him that when he does something wrong (which happened quite a bit), he was better off coming and telling me, rather than waiting for me to find it. So he came and found me and was crying, and told me what he had done—we walked over to the steps and there was a hole in the wall. I very calmly sent him to his room so I could figure out what to do. About ten minutes later, he came down and asked if he could get out of time-out. I said no, I had not decided yet what his punishment would be for punching the hole in the wall. I had him eat supper in his room, and he brought his plate down and asked again if he could come down. I said no, and then I came up with the perfect solution. He has low muscle tone in his hands and *hates* to write. So I went upstairs, with a notepad and a pencil, and told him he could get up and go play after he wrote a 100-word essay telling me how he was feeling when he punched the wall, what would have been a better way to have handled that situation, and why he wouldn't do it again. I have to say, I did get a ninety-eight-word essay. Now, there were quite a few repetitions—'I am so, so, so, so, so sorry'—but I still gave him credit for it. The writing works great for certain things. If he does something against a friend, I make him write a note of apology. He hates writing, but he does it, and we move on from there until the next time!"

In Appendix E, I have listed several excellent books that may help you in putting a behavior therapy program into place if you haven't done so already.

Play to the Child's Strengths

Behavior therapy helps you implement a careful consequence system and manage your child's misbehavior, but that doesn't necessarily mean it will create a positive self-image in your child, as this parent notes: "What is the most important thing a parent should do? Have a great sense of humor and don't get too lost in a bad moment. Always accentuate the positives in your child and try to downplay the annoying and negative as much as possible."

Remember, your child is much more likely to succeed as an adult if he gets lots of early encouragement and develops a sense of pride in some special area of ability—a lesson learned and applied by this parent:

> "Throughout Benjamin's life, we continually focused on his 'islands of competence' [in Hallowell's *Driven to Distraction*], and he never felt like a failure. Although he struggled in certain areas, he was always able to say, 'But I'm really good at _____.' [For him it was building, design, using a scientific calculator, working on the computer, etc.] I think that identifying these 'islands of competence' and then reinforcing and building on these strengths is one of the most essential things that parents and teachers can do for these children; self-esteem in the person with ADD can be very fragile. Also, positive motivation will go much farther than negative discipline techniques in shaping behavior in the ADD child."

That has certainly been my experience as well.

Schedule One-on-One Time

One thing you might try is to schedule a regular time with your child—just his time, no one else's—when you pursue an activity that your child likes and can help choose, and that you can enjoy together. I used to set up a regular one-on-one breakfast with each of my children, including with my son with ADHD. He also liked to go fishing, and I would take him on a fairly regular basis. Given his early difficulties, I found I always had to bite my lip to avoid my natural tendency to correct him every minute or two and to ignore low-level, only trivially problematic behaviors. Too much was at stake: We hadn't had a very good relationship for a while, and I knew I needed to reconnect. I made it my rule to use frequent praise for the things he was doing well and only very infrequent cautions, commands, and reprimands.

When Your Parenting Strategies and the Behavior Therapy Aren't Working

• *He's just not responding.* This happens, of course, but there's almost always a discoverable reason: Maybe you set a goal that doesn't meet the criteria of being clear, very specific, and achievable. Or the reward or consequence provides insufficient incentive. (See Appendix I for a list of possible rewards and ask for your child's input in choosing an alternative.) Or it will take the child so long to score a "success" that the reward's appeal recedes into the distance.

- *She "hates" the behavior program.* Look for several problems: Is your relationship strained, so that your daughter feels this is just a program to control or manipulate her, and she resents you? If so, work first on your relationship. In fact, a good relationship between you and your child is almost always a prerequisite for an effective behavior management program. Go back to the preceding sections on taking charge of your relationship.

Is it because she feels she *can't* succeed? Set lower goals: Shorten the period at the end of which success is measured, and reduce the number of behaviors that the child must acquire or eliminate, or some combination. By and large, she must be able to succeed about seventy percent of the time, or the program won't work.

- *You don't like the idea of bribing your child to behave appropriately.* First, understand that behavior therapy programs offer rewards, not bribes, and there is a difference. A bribe is something you give to someone who promises to do something in the future (e.g., you give your child something so that she *will* be good). A reward is something you give according to previously negotiated agreements, *after* the child has shown the behavior. Second, if you resent having to "pay" your child for meeting what seem like reasonable expectations, get over it. No one does anything without having some good reason to do so. You wouldn't go to work without getting paid, would you? Don't worry that you are teaching your child bad habits or teaching the wrong reasons to do the right thing. Couple the reward your child earns with your praise and expressions of love and pride in his accomplishment: In the long run, that is what will motivate him—if your relationship is strong.

- *Your child accuses you of cheating on delivering the rewards and has stopped cooperating.* Do you "cheat"? Have you been changing the rules? Some parents don't feel right about bestowing a reward on their child when, right after earning it, the child does something outrageous. You *must* follow through on delivering the reward, even if it sticks in your craw. A deal is a deal, and if you don't follow through, the consequences are usually much worse. Your child's resentment and sense of unfairness increases, and now you're really stuck. Follow through on all earned rewards.

If, however, you and your child disagree on the terms of the agreement, sit down and hash out the agreement again, and make sure you spell it all out in writing.

- *You just can't figure out why it's not working.* Have a heart-to-heart talk and ask your child why it is not working. What does she think would work better? Listen carefully and incorporate the input. If that leads nowhere, see an expert behavior therapist. Find one at *www.aabt.org*. Or ask an experienced parent for input and try it again.

- *You just forget to track the behavior and complete the chart.* If you find behavior programs too complicated to stick with the routine, ask your spouse or a close family friend or uncle to take this on—as long as it's someone who has frequent contact with the child and whom the child really likes. Also consider the possibility that you have ADHD as well. Get evaluated and treated if self-examination reveals that you have trouble concentrating and sticking with tasks in other areas, too.

Still Can't Seem to Improve Your Child's Behavior?: Seven Tips from Parents for Turning the Tide

When nothing seems to be working, consider the following possibilities:

1. *Increase your reinforcements of positive efforts.* "When you notice your child *trying* to do the things you are trying to help her with, let her *know* you notice and appreciate it."

    "Reward your child for even small accomplishments. I praise my son when he completes a chore on his own, or even when he sounds out words he has trouble with. You will find that rewarding them for the small things goes a long way with ADHD kids."

    Or, a useful rule of thumb from another parent: "Give five positives to every criticism when speaking to your child."

2. *If your approach has become far too punitive, get professional help.* "In preschool (Head Start) I got called several times saying my child was out of control. I thought they could have provided some type of diagnosis, but they never suggested ADHD. When things got way out of control and we were harshly punishing him, we were recommended to Parents Anonymous, an intensive parent support group, where you are reported for any type of child abuse but are also given wonderful tools to help avoid inflicting physical harm on a child."

3. *Be ready to be on the go with your child.* "Sitting in front of the TV is not helpful. Make sure you have many activities in mind that include lots of exercise, hands-on experiences."

    "It is important to accommodate the child's needs for extra activity, a multitude of projects at one time (try to not worry about a messy house; this too shall pass)."

4. *Remember your child's worries and other problems that may come with ADHD.* "For a long time, Rhonda had anxiety about riding in the car—she had tantrums or stomach problems and was terrified we would get lost. One day we did—very lost—at dusk in a freeway maze far from home. She became hysterical, so I said, 'We can do this. We can do anything if we don't give up.' I have since said that more times than I can count. One day I was exhausted, trying to help her get a major report together, and she reminded me, 'Mom, remember when you said we can do anything? We can if we don't give up.' My words finally sank in. Calm consistency is the key."

5. *Avoid overstimulating your child.* "I threw my son a surprise party for his eighth birthday and that whole thing backfired on me. It was horrible. He was horrible. The party was two to three hours, and it took me almost an hour and a half to figure him out and help him accept the whole concept of the surprise. I had to let him do his thing to get comfortable with the situation instead of forcing him to just have fun. It's hard."

6. *Don't ignore the little cues and hints about how your child is feeling.* "In 2002, my first-grade daughter began sneaking out of class, wandering off from our home, and hiding from us in public places. School officials were terrified that her safety was at risk, so they basically expelled her from her class. Their only solu-

tion was to put her back into kindergarten, where she could be fenced in and not 'escape.' In retrospect, something has occurred to me. Before she would 'escape' from home or school, she would give us little clues of her need for a change of scenery. But, as adults, we all too often ignore the hints and cues of children. 'Our timetable is supreme and since you're the child, you have to wait!' My daughter could feel her need to escape, and she tried to tell us."

7. *Switch gears to acknowledge that your child is becoming a teenager.* "This prompted me to write a book—*ADHD and Driving: A Guide for Parents*—sponsored by CHADD. I'd appreciate your giving the advice to parents that this book should be read when the child is around eleven or twelve. There is a lot that can be done to prepare these kids for driving that should be done *before* they get their learner's permit."

Or as advised by another parent, "We worked really hard with Kevin's doctor on educating Kevin about drugs and alcohol, and the impact they can have on a young person's life."

Making the Daily Household Routines Work for You

If you don't have a plan to address these issues, and if you don't convey this plan and your expectations to your spouse and children, household routines are going to be nonexistent, or they will all involve you doing the work—much too big a burden to carry for the next ten years or so. So let's start from what might be your reasonable expectations of others.

What You Should Expect from Your Household Routines

Help from Others

While it may seem like too much trouble to expect a young child, even a three-year-old, to help, if you don't start now, it will be harder (but not impossible) later. So regardless of what you have done in the past, let's set a new rule: Everyone in the family who can speak and understand simple requests is a part of your team to handle household chores. This is not a Holiday Inn, and you are not a maid or bellboy. Simple tasks, such as picking up, hanging up one's coat, putting books and schoolwork away, and caring for personal items is required for every family member. This includes your spouse, your child with ADHD, and all your other kids.

Time for Yourself

You deserve the freedom to pursue activities that are just for you, to recharge your batteries. We'll address this further when we discuss your personal life, a little later in this chapter. But this is certainly one big reason to make sure the household routines don't take up all your time.

Fairness and Respect—for Yourself and Other Family Members

Having and taking time for yourself also teaches important principles to your child with ADHD and to other family members, in that it models the idea that basic respect for others and teamwork are necessary parts of life. Don't avoid defending your own needs, because that will inadvertently teach your children that it's OK to walk on you. It's not. Ensuring that you get your own needs met, particularly when it means that others must give a little, teaches citizenship and fair play.

Parents sometimes make the mistake of making the entire family revolve around meeting the children's needs. While children do indeed have many needs and are somewhat more dependent on adults than adults are on children, it is still a two-way street. So for the long-term benefit of your children's character, you can and should insist that your children consider your needs, including your needs for your own activities, time alone, and their assistance in making that possible. Of course, the same rule must apply to other family members; you can and should expect your child with ADHD and siblings to respect the rights and needs of each other.

Understanding and appreciation are rarely forthcoming from children, however, so don't expect too much from your children. Yes, you have the right to expect and must insist on fairness from your children, but don't expect them to be happy about it—after all, they're *kids* and don't yet have the emotional maturity to respond that way. So they may try to make you feel guilty, and they may complain (that's their job, and the very definition of being childish and immature), but your job as a parent is to stick to your guns and insist on what is needed (your job is to teach them and to model mature behavior for them), even when they squawk (which they always will).

Some Modest Amount of Routine and Predictability to Life

Life with a child with ADHD is not easy, but it can be rewarding, and you—and every parent—can learn to adapt and make things work for you. Patience is important, because learning what works for you and your family takes a bit of time. Yes, you will have to adjust your expectations, but you can still have expectations. It's just that your expectations have to be tempered by your flexibility and willingness to "drop back and punt" from time to time when the battles seem too great. I don't know who said it, but the adage "Consistency is the hobgoblin of little minds" is important to remember. Sometimes parents get worried that if they make an exception or aren't perfectly consistent every time, they will teach the child bad habits. In fact, making exceptions and allowing some variations in routines is fine, as long as you make clear that they are exceptions and your reasons are sensible and conveyed to your child. Much better that you show that you can think on your feet, respond to changing circumstances, than to stick to some principle that in the long run won't make much difference. As an example, with my own children, we have usually had routines such as doing homework right after school. But my wife discovered that this principle did not in fact work very well with our son with ADHD, who came home tense and wound up. So she wisely decided to let him unwind after school, get a snack, and play for a while in the backyard, before focusing him on getting his homework done. This may not work for every child with ADHD, but it did for him—and for us.

Good Times, Bad Times

Yes, there will be lots of good times. And you will probably have more than your share of bad times, too, but there is hope for every child and every parent of a child with ADHD. Most children with ADHD can be helped to have full, productive, happy lives. The important thing is that you keep your eyes on the horizon. Don't be too discouraged by any setback, whether it lasts just a day, a month, or a year. Your child's ultimate outcomes are built slowly over time, and setbacks, regardless of how bad they seem right when they are happening, are almost always temporary. What will make a bigger difference than any setback will be your optimism and the hope that you hold in your heart and convey to your child, so that she too can feel it, believe it, and ultimately realize it.

Play as Well as Work

All work and no play makes . . . everyone cranky! If families were meant only to clothe, feed, and house kids, orphanages or youth hostels would be much cheaper. Remember, your home should be a safe haven, a sanctuary where adults and children can bond, can feel understood and accepted by each other (at least sometimes!), where family members can relax and have fun, and be spontaneous. So in all of the efforts you expend on assisting your child with ADHD, relax and have fun together. Refer back to the principles in Chapter 2: Many of these are based on realism, compassion, and balance. When we apply these at home, they can make living there a lot happier.

If you find you are never having good times together, you have a critical problem that must be addressed as quickly as possible. If my ideas under "Having Some Fun" on page 182 don't work, bring it up with your doctor and consider asking for a referral to a therapist.

Taking Charge: How to Get What You Need at Home

How can you get what you expect, so that your home operates smoothly, with minimal conflict, while also remaining a place that everyone looks forward to coming back to? Here, a little planning and organization—and also lots of compassion and love—can go a long way to getting your expectations met.

Home Organization Systems

To create some helpful routines, it will be useful for you to learn as much as you can about home organization systems and strategies for making household routines. In our own family, we read several books on household management (see Appendix E for my suggestions) and along the way picked up a number of useful tips. So, for example, we decided early on to teach the children the habit of picking up toys after playing. This became a routine before bedtime, where we would have a little race or fun contest where we all worked together to put the toys away, seeing how rapidly we could get it done or who could do the most toys. We did this because we thought it would be useful for the children (including the child with ADHD) to learn such habits.

Another strategy was to develop the habit of children making their beds before leaving for school. To avoid hassles, we found it worked best to put such activities on a point chart, allowing all of the children (including the child with ADHD) to make points to earn some favored treat or activity. Although we started this program principally for our child with ADHD, the other children wanted to be able to win prizes too, so what the heck! Even now we tend to set up little goal charts, and my kids (including my son with ADHD) now do them for themselves as a goal-setting strategy and will even put me on a chart to monitor my weight or to do regular exercise.

Another strategy for household routines that we found useful was "Saturday chores." Suzy drew up a list of five or six different routine household chores (e.g., vacuuming, emptying trash, sweeping the floors, cleaning the bathrooms, etc.), writing the complete description of what each job entailed on index cards. Children got to rotate which job they did on a regular basis. We had a similar strategy for daily dishes: Each child had to pick a day of the week to wash the dishes. Children age eight or older were taught to do them on their own, and even when our children were ages four to seven, they learned to assist us or one of the older ones.

And then there was "the dreaded clothes bag." Suzy found that she was often picking up the kids' clothes that were strewn about the house, so she got a tip from one book to confiscate such clothing items, putting them in a bag. A child who wanted that item back would have to draw a job (marked on little pieces of paper) from the "job jar." In the job jar, she had put all kinds of household chores that needed to be done, in addition to the Saturday chores. This strategy worked particularly well with preteens and teens, who often had particular favorite clothes items.

Should the child with ADHD be asked to do chores? Of course. At what age? In my experience, at the same age as other kids would be, as a general rule. We started all of our kids with picking up their toys right before bedtime as early as age two or three. But we did it together, talking about it, making it into a game, having a race, and so on. Helping your child with ADHD assume responsibility is doubly important if there is more than one kid in the family; otherwise, it will stoke anger and jealousy if the child with ADHD always seems to get off easy. What this means is that he or she will still have to bear reasonably similar responsibilities, but *you* will have to offer extra support, to assist him or her in taking that responsibility.

Each family is different, so you'll have to ask yourself, what's really important for you? What gets most under your skin? Maybe it's the empty orange juice container left in the fridge or the muddy shoes tracked into the kitchen, or things left around that you feel like you have to follow around and pick up. Or the issue might not be housekeeping-related at all, but the amount of driving kids around you have to do, or shopping, or paying bills. How might these tasks be divvied up, or your burdens lessened? How about setting some limits or rules about no more than one or two extracurricular activities per week? Or the requirement that you'll drive once a week to the soccer practice, also taking your child's friends to it, but that the other two times are for the other parents? Or for your spouse? Or, if your child is old enough, for him or her to arrange his own ride? Remember, don't feel guilty about setting limits. As much as possible, your child needs a rested, patient, unharried parent.

Extra Household Help

One strategy that you might consider if you can afford it is to get some extra household help. This needn't be a big deal, but even once every other week can make a difference, and you don't need to feel guilty about this. Often there are some bigger tasks that may be important to you but you just never seem to get time for, such as cleaning the floors or polishing the furniture. Your tasks of parenting are the most important areas to spend your energy, so if you can afford it, try this one out.

You may have other options available to you as well, even if you can't afford to pay someone: For example, have your friend or sister, the neat freak, do your weekly cleaning if you, the enthusiastic cook, will fill her freezer with pasta sauces and soups. Can you think of others?

Family Planning

No, not *that* kind of family planning! Here I mean scheduling a weekly meeting with everyone where you map out a family plan. This needs to be done in such a way that parents and children all feel like they have their say in what needs to be talked about. If there is only one child, this is very possible, but keep it balanced, so that the child doesn't feel double-teamed or that it is all about him. What could be on the table for discussion that all of you can meaningfully talk over and problem-solve? For example, a family meeting is the right format for discussing new rules or routines. If someone is planning a special household project, such as putting in new shelves, a family meeting could be a good place to see how others might be involved or coordinate preparation and cleanup.

To make this meeting part of your weekly routine, try to find a time when everyone is usually home, perhaps a weeknight or a Sunday evening. Mom or Dad might conduct the meeting, with a clear agenda mapped out. Children's opinions should be encouraged and sought, but remember, a family is not a democracy. In the long run, parents have to make major decisions, but as your children get older, more and more of the decisions that affect them will be made by joint consultation, discussion, and compromise before a final agreement is reached. And with activities within their own sphere of competence, you will want to give even young children increasing opportunities to make their own decisions, perhaps with your input.

The weekly planning meeting might also be used to coordinate schedules, discuss upcoming events, congratulate family members for special accomplishments made during the week, make weekly chore assignments, discuss roles and responsibilities, and encourage children to talk about feelings or family matters. Making a fun family game and a snack or dessert a part of such a meeting can keep everyone enthused and looking forward to such meetings.

Having Some Fun

"Make sure they have time to be kids."

That's a very important reminder from a very wise parent. Your child with ADHD can end up feeling like life is so regimented, and every little task requires such strict protocol from him, that all of the joy can be sucked out of childhood. If things like home organization, point charts, and so on, are increasing conflict, it's time to get a professional consultation and debug the strategy.

Also, be sure to go out of your way and schedule fun times. Sometimes they won't happen unless you provide the time and space for them in the family calendar. Solicit your child's ideas for the best ways to have fun together and then plan them together. During the activity, avoid criticism, focusing as much on doing the thing that you and your child enjoy together. So, for example, if your child enjoys fishing, do that. Or video games? Play some together. I bought my son a particular video game but also stipulated that it could be played only when he and I worked on it together. I really was pleased then when he sought me out so we could play together.

What to Do When Household Routines Fall Apart

Let's face it: The real world (not just your home) is a pretty messy place. So what do you do when you are *still* the only one who does any work around the place? Or how about when things are always chaotic: You've tried everything, but you can't seem to make any system work? And if things are still disorganized? Or if everybody's so sick of being organized that you're all constantly on edge and ready to snap? Here are some questions to ask yourself:

• *Is it time to reevaluate your expectations?* Do they need to be lowered? Remember, you have plenty of battles to fight, and it may be that keeping the house as clean as you or others might seem to expect is asking a bit too much at this point. Simply getting your child to school on time, helping him get homework done, keeping sibling rivalry down to a dull roar, and handling your own job on the side are all significant achievements in and of themselves. And who wants their gravestone or obituary to say at the top of their list of accomplishments, "Most important, she kept a clean house"? Refer to the principles in Chapter 2, and to your action plan: Is the clean house one of your top priorities?

• *Is this the most important battle to fight?* Is it the right time to fight it? In making the system work for your child with ADHD, you have lots of areas to tackle, and your personal energy is needed in many places. Are household routines and chores really an important issue right now? *The* most important issue? Or is reconnecting as a family and just doing something fun together likely to refuel you for the coming week more than the cleanest and neatest house could possibly do?

- *Are you fully "armed and ready" for this battle?* Have you done sufficient reading to learn about strategies for household management? If not, this may be a good time for you to take a strategic step back, learn more about various household management ideas, and wait until you're sure you have sufficient supplies and lots of ammo to tackle the problem. Are there some good strategies there that you haven't tried?

- *Do you have everyone's support in implementing the plan, including that of your spouse?* If not, you may need to reevaluate your options. Do you need to compromise more and set somewhat different goals that others can support? It's hard to pull this off all if the other adults in the home aren't pulling with you.

- *Are communications clear?* Did you implement your new household management strategy through clear communication with all parties involved, with expectations written out so there was no room for being second-guessed about what the expectations really are? Are house rules, tasks, assignments, and consequences written down and posted where others can see them? Would you find a white board with dry erase markers helpful, perhaps posted close to the refrigerator or by the phone?

- *Have you discussed it with a friend?* Everyone—I mean everyone who has one or more children—has had to learn certain household management techniques. There's lots of wisdom out there, and no one is born knowing how to do it. Lots of this is learned through trial and error. Talk with your friends about this. What has worked for them? What advice would they give you?

- *Are there any "teeth" to your plan?* Are there "consequences" when someone does not pull his own weight or do her part? If not, this is not going to work. If you feel you just can't put the consequences in place, this is not the right time to do this. You need to store up energy and/or get advice and help from others so that you implement that part of the overall household management strategy. It's not one you can delegate.

- *Time to discuss it with your doctor?* Sometimes we can be personally overwhelmed, which in turn makes it harder to be organized and to implement organizational systems. In particular, this can happen when adults become discouraged, demoralized, or depressed. Or if we ourselves have enough ADHD traits that organizational issues are difficult. So could you be depressed, or might you have ADHD? Talk this one over candidly with your doctor.

- *Should you get some professional assistance?* "Get an ADHD coach who works with parents of children with ADHD," strongly encourages one parent. One of the great sources of support for adults is that there are now many professional "coaches" out there who can be hired on an hourly basis to come in and help you get organized. Coaches can be found through any of the many major ADHD organizations, such as CHADD or ADDA, and the programs at the yearly meetings of these associations are chock-full of coaches and other similar persons with expertise in these areas.

- *How about a maid?* If you didn't like this idea before, is it time to reconsider it? Just a bit of extra help, even once a month, may make a great deal of difference to your peace of mind if this issue continues to weigh on you.

• *Is it time to go "on strike"?* If you feel that you are not making headway with your family members and that you are still more like the hired help than management, is it time to go on strike? Talk this one over with a couple of friends and get their advice before taking this step. But a one- or two-day strike without meals, laundry, or shuttle service can get a lot of attention. You have to watch it with this, though. I have a friend who once left her husband and daughter a note saying that if they didn't start cleaning out the cat box as they *swore* they would before she agreed to get a kitten, she was going to stop cooking all the meals. She had really had it with unfulfilled requests to clean the litter regularly. Her daughter's reaction totally stunned her: She burst into tears and wailed, "But how am I going to eat dinner?" She was only six, and it never occurred to her mother that in a child's limited world, if the mother didn't cook dinner for her, she'd actually starve!

EXERCISE 1

How to Get Your Family to Cooperate with Routines . . . When Nothing Has Worked Before

Role-play this scenario with a friend. Have him or her take the role of your child and spouse, while you play yourself. Encourage your friend to come up with a variety of objections in the role of the children, so that you can prepare to respond to whatever the kids come up with when you use this strategy in real life.

Once you're ready to do this with your actual kids, call a family powwow, where both your spouse and your child(ren) are present. Ahead of time, you and your spouse must agree on this plan. If not, have the powwow with your spouse alone, until you're in agreement.

YOU: Things are going to change around here. I am doing all of the picking up, cleaning, cooking, washing, and driving.

SPOUSE (OR YOU, IF YOU ARE SINGLE): That's right. It's not been fair for your mother (me), or even good for you kids. It's teaching you bad habits. So as of today, things will be different.

YOU OR SPOUSE: We have put ten chores in this bottle. Everyone gets to draw two out of the bottle. These must be done each week, every Saturday, before you play or go out. If you do each of your chores on time and without complaining, you will get to earn three points for each job. If I have to remind or nag you, then you'll just get two points. If you complain, just one point per job. Points count for rewards that you can get.

SPOUSE OR YOU: We're going to let each of you children pick the rewards you most want, as long as it's not too expensive. Then we'll together decide how many points it's worth (*see Appendix I for ideas about rewards*). Then when you've earned the points, we'll go together and get that reward.

CHILD(REN): Why do we have to do that? Johnny doesn't have to do anything, and his family has a maid do all the chores.

YOU OR SPOUSE: What Johnny's family does is fine for Johnny's family. This is what our family does. It's important for you kids to learn this. I know it's new, but you'll get used to it. And if you work quickly, you'll find that the jobs take only about half an hour. If you dawdle, it'll take you all day. But the jobs need to be done.

SPOUSE OR YOU: It's not fair that your mother (father) does all of these things, and everyone needs to do their part around here. I'm doing some chores too!

CHILD(REN): It's not fair. No one else in my school has to do chores!

YOU OR SPOUSE: Life isn't always fair. But it's most important that everyone learn to help out. You'll find it's not so bad. But remember, it's important to try to have a good attitude and not complain, so you'll be able to make points more quickly. Now, let's look over the reward list. What rewards do you think you want to work for?

Making Your Home Relationships Work for You

"It takes an entire family to deal with a child with ADHD. Everyone has to come to terms with the fact that things have to adjust to the child."

You, just like your child, need people who are in your corner and rooting for you. For most of us, this means the home front. Our spouse and children, although they consume a lot of energy, should also give something back that helps and sustains us. If not, why are we doing this? It should not be just a chore or simply a matter of waiting until all the kids are grown and out of the house. That would be a long wait. And if there are no payoffs now, there probably won't be any later. So we must make sure the odds are fixed and we can get some short-term payoffs. The surest way to fix the odds? You must *have* and *hold* some clear expectations for others in the home.

What You Should Expect from Your Spouse and Children

From Your Spouse . . .

• *Not to be blamed for your child's difficulties.* "I am divorced and have a rocky relationship with my ex," said one mother. "He often blames me for everything, including Jonathan's ADHD and associated problems. We had *many* fights over the issue early on. Over the years (it has been seven years since the initial diagnosis), he has become more rational about the matter, but he still blames me for everything." Sometimes one parent (usually the father) assumes that because the child with ADHD behaves better for him than for the other parent, this means that the other parent is just not a good disciplinarian or is too much of a pushover with the child. This notion is almost always incorrect and fails to account for the fact that children with ADHD have highly variable behavior. Yes, they may *temporarily* respond to a father's gruff command or foreboding physical presence, but if that same father had to do all of the parenting, day in and day out, the novelty of the gruff command and physical presence would wear off, and the child would eventually show just as many behavioral difficulties and noncompliance as with the parent he spent more time with (even in today's society, this is still usually the mother). And when one parent "blows in" and barks a command to the child, all the while subtly blaming the other parent for not being more like him, strong negative forces begin to operate on the marital relationship. "It was ruining my marriage" is not an uncommon assessment of how this can turn out. Said one mom: "My husband blames *me* for our son's problems. Somehow I am not strict enough. He comes in like gangbusters, not understanding what Justin is going through, and makes things even worse by threats and punishments. And then I have to deal with my son's emotional wreckage for the next two days. I doubt myself and wonder if my husband is right, though. As a couple, we are not playing from the same sheet of music . . . we're probably not in the same orchestra. I'm not sure, but that is probably contributing to the situation too." If you and your spouse have discussed this and it remains an issue, it's worth seeking marriage counseling.

• *Understanding and support.* If you are reading this book, chances are you are on the front lines doing more of the daily battles than your spouse. And as you know, it's hard work, extremely taxing emotionally, and as a result much harder than most jobs. If your spouse has any doubts about this, it's time for you to take a few days or up to a week off, leaving your spouse in charge. If your spouse has any doubts, most of them will be gone by the time you return.

"I am divorced from my child's father for thirteen years now," one mother told me, "but he has chosen not to deal with his daughter's needs. He has chosen not to educate himself on the condition and sees her as little as possible due to her negativity toward his new family and stepchildren. As far as my husband of twelve years goes, we have worked on this together since the day we discovered there was a problem. It has been difficult at times, but we relied on each other in the low times to keep each other motivated when we felt like giving up. His support has made all the difference." Not getting support and understanding from your spouse in handling your child's ADHD difficulties can be a serious problem and may wreak havoc over the long term in a marriage, generating resentment, arguments, and increasing emotional distance. Don't let this one fester; instead, make it an issue for discussion and problem solving early on, rather than later, after it has clogged up your communication channels.

• *Sharing responsibility.* You and your spouse, as well as your older children, must share in the various responsibilities for running the household. If it is all on your back, and you find yourself always the one picking up the slack, it's time to evaluate and adjust roles and patterns. In the long run, in terms of helping each other out, a good marriage should be approximately fifty–fifty, but in the short run, it may be seventy–thirty or even twenty–eighty. If one parent has an illness, or a particularly bad time at work, the other may carry more of the burden—"in sickness and in health." So if you are bearing more of the burden, this has to be acknowledged, and there has to be trust and mutual support that it will balance out over time. But if marriage partners are busy counting who did what, and who owes whom how much, something is awry. Trust and genuine sharing of responsibilities cannot be handled like legal contracts, and if a marriage is headed in that direction, its time to get some counseling.

- *Thanks and appreciation.* You need and deserve thanks and appreciation for all you do. Don't expect your spouse to read your mind on this one. Spouses—we men in particular—are not especially sensitive creatures, and we need to have these issues pointed out from time to time. So don't fall into the common trap of thinking "If she *really* cared, then she would know that . . ." Tell her what you need. Communicating your needs, including your needs for appreciation, is your responsibility. It is the other partner's responsibility to provide it. But mind-reading was not in the marriage vows. Nonetheless, because misunderstandings can so frequently arise when a family is under stress, it might be a good rule of thumb to look actively for ways to show each other your appreciation.

- *Time to get away by yourselves.* "We realized it was either we have a date night once a week, or we go to a marriage counselor. A date night is less expensive and more fun." So said one father with a twinkle in his eye. For a marriage to survive the stress of having a child with ADHD, you'll need time to get away together by yourselves. A weekly outing or date, or even just a regular walk together is critical to keeping this relationship intact. And you must talk about things other than your child. What interests did you share when you got married? What are each other's interests and hobbies? What happened in your spouse's day that made him happy? Or sad? What went well? What was the hardest thing about her day? This needs to be shared in a two-way fashion. It's good for you to ask these questions and listen, but don't forget to ask for and expect the same in return.

Of course there are practical matters to consider: "I have concerns about obtaining a babysitter," one mother said. "How can I choose someone to handle the extremes in behavior? So I just don't go out." There are other options, however: How about trading out babysitting with another parent whose child has similar problems? Or seeking a volunteer through your church? Or contacting respite services from your local agencies, talked about in Chapter 4 under "Tangible Supports."

From Your Other Kids . . .

Here's a good sample of the types of problems you are likely experiencing:

> "My son is verbally aggressive and provocative to his older sister, and I feel angry many days that he vents his frustrations on her. I do a lot to help her understand her brother's difficulties, and I frequently try to head off his verbal attacks on her or stop him after the first utterance. I feel super vigilant when the two of them are in a room together, waiting for the inevitable sparring to begin. His sister is actually academically gifted, and he is terribly jealous of her. She's a friendly, outgoing girl with many friends. She handles him well but sometimes erupts out of frustration. I just take it one day at a time."

> "My daughter has also been affected. She is a year younger than him—and many times I see her taking a motherly role with him. She tends to be protective of

him . . . but at the same time, she gets totally frustrated with him. She has commented that she gets tired of his ADD and the way *she* has to deal with it, too."

"My husband and I have been married for eighteen years. This has definitely put a strain on our marriage. I find myself being more lenient toward my son versus my daughter. This in turn makes it hard for my daughter to accept her brother as an equal."

What are some strategies that you can employ to problem-solve these issues?

• *Doing a regular chore that contributes to the overall family good.* The problem here, of course, is that you must yourself get organized and follow through with these requests and monitor your child's completion of tasks, including walking him through the task with gentle but persistent insistence. Lots of praise for the child's efforts, and perhaps using a behavior program to reinforce his completion of assigned tasks may help. Inconsistency will bite you here and undermine your plans or assignments. You may think it's more trouble than it's worth, and you just go ahead and do it anyway. Not a good idea. You lose the chance to teach responsibility, then you get more resentful that everything depends on you and that you have to do all the work!

• *Managing their own "stuff."* Each child should be responsible for, take care of, and put away his or her own toys, clothes, books, and other belongings. For young children, you'll have to do it side by side with them until they learn that it is really expected and they can't wait you out. Couple this with some of the strategies given earlier or a simple behavioral program for each child.

• *Learning and obeying house rules.* Have you made them clear? Are they written down and posted? Are they discussed on a regular basis, particularly when there are infractions? Do you and your spouse follow them as well? Do you have a family pow-wow to rediscuss them and problem-solve, with kids' input if they aren't following them, seeking their input as to why and what might be possible solutions?

• *Personal hygiene.* Is there a set time and routine for these activities, such as brushing teeth *before* story time for younger children? Getting dressed before coming downstairs and having breakfast? Getting pajamas on before dessert or turning on the TV? There are a thousand variations on this theme, all using the "before" rule. This works well, but be consistent rather than on and off. Even if you're tired, it is worth the extra effort. You're teaching organizational habits that will reduce your workload in the long run.

• *Getting along with siblings.* Don't assume this will just happen. In fact, it won't. It will be a message that you must repeat again and again. Just go with it, be patient, and understand that that is how kids learn—repeated reminders over time, consistent praise and rewards for doing it, regular consequences, without your getting too upset when they don't. All kids fight, all kids pick on each other. And the kids you think are blameless or just the victims usually aren't; in fact, they often find sneaky ways to retaliate that escape your notice. If things continue to be quite bad or get worse and threaten children's safety and your sanity, consider a joint reward system, where you reward both children together when they get along, and reward neither when they don't, even if you think only one of them is to blame. In the long run, this will keep them from setting each other up for punishment or failure and strengthen sibling relationships and adult friendships. If things are really bad or physically dangerous, get professional help.

Taking Charge: How to Get What You Need from Your Relationships

Convey Clear Expectations and Rules

Remember, you are in this for the long run. If each day is impossible, adjustments must be made, and all must make some accommodations, including accommodations for you. Others are responsible for meeting at least some of your needs, but you are responsible for communicating your needs and expectations. Don't fall into the trap of feeling guilty for making demands on others. But, likewise, don't lay a guilt trip on others (e.g., "If only you knew how much I sacrifice for you . . .").

Work to Create a Positive Climate

This is easily done with positive comments, small praises, whether they be for your spouse or for your children. It is all too easy to get caught up in the habit of noticing only negative behaviors and missing or ignoring when people (adults or children) do something right. As we like to say to parents about comments to children, "Catch them being *good!*" As a general rule, positive comments should outnumber negative or critical comments four to one. Don't sweat the small stuff. If there is a negative climate—one of criticism or blame—in the home, all of the other good efforts will often not make much of a difference in the long run.

Chill Out

Maybe it's not your problem . . . it's theirs. So don't expend a lot of time and energy on getting people to change things that aren't likely to change. Figure out what is really important and insist on that. And when the other stuff gets under your skin, take a walk. Count to ten. Count to ten again . . . and again. Talk to a friend. Have your nails done. Write a letter or e-mail you've been postponing.

What to Do When There Is Constant Tension between You and Your Spouse or between Your Child with ADHD and Siblings

- *Talk about it!* "We were told our other son acts out because all the attention was on our other child. He says he often also wants to move out (he is fourteen). He seems to grin and bear it, but when we have a talk about it, he tells me it is unbearable." It's critical that you ask your other kids outright how they feel about having a sibling with ADHD. Don't expect that you can make all the problems go away, of course, but letting your child share his feelings will allow you to be supportive and encouraging; then, using that information, cut him some extra slack from time to time, when the pressure seems to be getting to him.

• *Use behavioral programs for dealing with sibling relationship problems.* Sometimes the biggest challenges may come from fighting between your child with ADHD and your other children. In our own family, we often found it most useful to use behavioral charts not just for our child with ADHD but for the other children as well. Yes, your child with ADHD may be more likely to be the provocateur, but this is not always the case, as I once found out: It seemed to me that my son with ADHD was always picking on his younger brother. In fact, we had witnessed it many times. But what we did not realize, at least for a period of months or years, was that the younger child, Jonathan, had found clever ways to retaliate against his older brother David with ADHD: In fact, the fights were not infrequently started by Jonathan, who by age five had found out that by crying as if he had been hit by David, he could get his older brother in trouble with Mom and Dad—a pretty cool trick! Only when we discovered this (and began to hold them jointly responsible for getting along) did we turn the corner on the sibling fighting that always *seemed* to be precipitated by the child with ADHD. Wrong.

In our family, we ended up having several star charts going at any given time, most often for the child with ADHD, but also sometimes for another child, to learn to deal with his or her end of some sibling squabble: perhaps not to yell when provoked or to learn to negotiate and problem-solve.

• *Get professional help for family members who need it.* When a sibling without ADHD is tormented by one with ADHD, and also watches conflict develop between parents because of the child's ADHD, troublesome feelings about the child with ADHD can definitely develop. How are these kids supposed to handle these uncomfortable feelings, especially when Mom and Dad are simply too busy to take charge? As one parent pointed out ruefully, "Health insurance does not pay for counseling for the other kids." In fact, almost all insurance companies will pay for what are called "collateral visits," where other family members can be seen as a means of assisting the primary patient. In addition, if the parents and/or siblings have their own difficulties, there will be similar coverage within that insurance program for each family member, based on them receiving their own diagnosis.

• *Investigate family therapy.* Family therapy is not effective as a treatment for ADHD per se, so don't go there. However, it can be very helpful when the family has lots of communication problems, when things are in perpetual chaos, and/or when roles and responsibilities seem confused or unfair. Family therapy can be stressful, so talk with friends who have been through family therapy and get their input as to what therapists have been helpful.

• *Marriage counseling.* Have you considered marriage counseling? You may want to raise this issue with your spouse. Sometimes a pastor, priest, or rabbi can do this, if you both are of the same religious persuasion. Also, professionally trained and licensed marriage counselors are available in pretty much every locale. Sometimes it may be something a social worker, psychologist, or psychiatrist does, but you'll have to ask around. Check with your doctor, who will likely know a few names. And as with family therapy, don't go into this blind. Find someone you both can trust. Talk with friends who have been through marriage counseling, and see whether there is anyone they can recommend. It can be stressful, but if the marriage relationship is in a tailspin, don't wait until it is too late to recover.

• *Talk with a friend and unwind.* Remember, all of your needs cannot be met at home, and you need other places to recharge your batteries. Do you have one or more friends you can relate to and confide in? If not, it's time to make these connections, whether at work, at church/synagogue, at the day care center, or somewhere else.

• *Step back and reevaluate.* If you have tried a host of options, and things are still not making sense, what's going on? Could you or your spouse be depressed? Might there be substance use problems or ADHD in either of you? If you or your child's other parent has ADHD or another problem, it can add an enormous burden to the demands of parenting a child with ADHD. And all of your good efforts and interventions may be of relatively little consequence if you don't attend to this problem of your own. If you are uncertain about whether something is wrong, speak with your doctor and get his input and advice about next steps.

Parents' Top Ten: How to Keep Peace in the Home and Happiness in the Family with ADHD

1. *Make sure you get away by yourself.* "We did things as a family, but we made sure that each of us had time away—my husband went on a two-week hunting trip; I went to flower shows or on shopping trips."
   "Take separate vacations from them even if it is only for two hours."

2. *Take time out for your marriage.* "We make sure we go on dates at least every other week and take a long weekend for ourselves about every six months."

3. *Put your child on a schedule and try to keep things as consistent as possible.* "The best advice I ever got," said one mother. For a child who gets very anxious about little things, this might translate as "remaining calm and patient, making everything as visual as possible for him, and sticking to a schedule."

4. *Offer your child all the love and patience you can muster.* One parent said that the best advice she ever got was "to draw upon the strength of my own personal religious beliefs" in striving to do this.

5. *Be creative.* Why? "No discipline strategy lasts for long," in the words of one wise parent.

6. *Act like Mr. Rogers.* "One day," a mother explained, "someone told me that the one and only genius with kids is Mr. Rogers. He is soft-spoken, very calm, and kids usually love him. So one day this person told me to try the Mr. Rogers attitude and see how our son would react to it. It was amazing. I kept my cool even though it's very hard, because our son is a high-strung, very stubborn little person. But I knew that if I lowered my level of tension, his would automatically follow. And it did. The biggest challenge for us is the fact that he is very honest and, whatever comes out of his mouth, you had better be ready. Especially in public."

(cont.)

---

7. *Find balance.* "Provide a firm but warm family environment."
8. *Journal your feelings.* A good way, said one parent, to "deal with the anger that comes from learning your child has ADHD and then the anger and frustration that comes with dealing with an ADHD child."
9. *The single most important thing we as parents can do is to create a refuge.* A clean, simple home filled with books, music, pets, and delicious food," said one parent.
10. *Find ways for your child to succeed.* "As important at home as it is at school, making your child feel successful can ease the child's irritation, head off sibling rivalry, and contribute to tranquillity."

A final word from one smart parent: "In some ways, our son has made our marriage stronger—we had to talk about everything! We had to share the burden of the crises that were almost an everyday occurrence. It seemed when one of us had had it the other would take over and vice versa. The doctor kept telling us that these kids often caused marital discord, so we took extra care not to let him get between us."

EXERCISE 2

How to Get Your Spouse to Stop Blaming You and Assume More Responsibility for Your Child's Care

Role-play this scenario with a friend. Have him or her play your spouse, while you play yourself. Then switch roles and do it again. My comments to you are in *italics.*

SPOUSE: You've just got to be stricter with [child's name]. He doesn't misbehave when he's with me. [*Watch out; this is called* blame.]

YOU: You are gone at work all day, and you don't have to pick up the pieces when [child's name] comes home discouraged and unhappy. Just being "strict" when he comes home backfires. I've tried that, and it only makes him feel worse. The issue is that he needs some one-on-one time to get his homework done, and I'm too exhausted to do all of it. I need you to help out with that when you come home. [*Good! Stick to your guns. Don't go ballistic; just stay the course.*]

SPOUSE: But I'm tired too. I've had a long day. How can you expect me to do that after a full day? [*Another guilt-trip attempt. But you now see it coming.*]

YOU: We have both had full days. The issue is that unless we both work together and give the same messages to him, it ends up being just a mother–son battle, which is not good for the mother–son, nor for our relationship. [*Nice logic, nice and steady argument. Keep it up!*]

SPOUSE: But you are home all day, and you've had plenty of time to relax. [*Wow! She/he's really pulling out the big guns. Don't let it faze you.*]

YOU: We can trade roles anytime you want. But we're in this together, and the issue here is that your son needs you. And for this, *I* need you, too. We can set a time, say from 7:30 to 8:30 every night, so you'll be able to plan for it. It's his math that is most needed, and the area I don't know. [*Nice recovery.*]

SPOUSE: I can't believe you're asking me to do this. You know how hard my work is. [*Last attempt at the guilt trip?*]

YOU: I know your day is stressful. But it's much easier to deal with clients than with your own son. If you don't believe me, you just try it. At any rate, we need to share this responsibility more. I need you to do this. I'd like to start tomorrow night. Besides, I have a PTA meeting then . . . unless you'd rather go, and I'll do the homework? [*Great strategy. You even have another child-relevant obligation, and either way, you're beginning to shift part of the responsibility!*]

SPOUSE: (*Silence.*) [*This is OK. You made your point, and you stuck to your guns. Silence for a few hours, even days is OK, but you must thicken your skin and stick to your guns. Much more than this single point is at stake. It's also your own mental health, as well as the balance of fairness in your marriage.*]

Making Your Personal Life Work for You

You will be happier and more relaxed if you feel good about yourself. And a happier you is going to be more able to respond to others, including your child with ADHD, when the chips are down. All of us are like automobiles: We can go and go, but eventually we have to refill our gas tanks. When we feel overstressed and irritable—something that happens to all of us—our tempers flare, and we may end up doing or saying things that we regret. This is a part of life, but it is a part of life we want to minimize if at all possible, since it tends to make things worse and add to our other burdens and challenges.

You owe it to yourself to take care of yourself. Care, compassion, and concern are things you owe yourself, as well as the rest of the family.

What You Should (and Should Not) Expect from Yourself

Human Error

"The hardest thing for me was that—even before my son experienced the difficulties associated with ADHD—I had developed defensiveness about my own behavior (extreme disorganization and randomness, which I attributed to 'creativity')—and I had been influenced by negative information concerning ADHD." Some parents, like the one quoted at the beginning of this chapter, end up hating themselves for their reaction to the stresses of raising a child with ADHD. Be patient and tolerant with yourself. You must like yourself if you want others to like you. While you cannot always count on others to appreciate what you do, you must value it. With some embarrassment, I recall the time in my less wise days of youth and early marriage when I was pressuring my wife to go out and get a job or advanced degree, when she was home spending time with our (at that time) three children. At one point, she figuratively grabbed me by the collar and said in effect (my translation; she would disavow ever using such strong language):

> "Listen, buster: it is because of *my* support at home that you get to spend long hours away at work, building a successful career. When I am ready—and when I think the kids are ready—for me to go out and get a job, I will. But in the meantime, I am doing something very valuable for *our* children. So don't tell me that I should go out and get a job, just so I can fit your image of 'the professional wife.' Any questions?"

When Suzy put her foot down (on top of mine), it was clear that she, first and foremost, valued what she was doing, even when I wasn't fully supportive. I am much more supportive now, but she weathered my lack of full support because her own internal compass about what was important to her kept a steady course. So remember, what is important to you *is* important to you, even when others don't always appreciate it. Hang on to it.

Likewise, forgive yourself for small foibles. Remember, you're going to make mistakes along the way. At times you will "blow it" with your child. You may lose your temper, be too harsh, or give in when you ought to be firm. We all do. So mistakes are part of the game. The important thing is not that you don't make mistakes but that you recognize them and, when appropriate, apologize for them.

Always remember that you have the right to forgive yourself for being human: None of us are perfect parents. . . . We don't come with parent genes, we learn through experiences, talking with others, and so on. So, why should we expect that we can parent kids with these challenges without help?

What to do when your human frailty rises to the surface? Find help and join a support group or get therapy.

The Ability to Cut Others a Bit of Slack

Whether it's your child with ADHD or another family member, it's best to assume that your family's intentions are to do the right thing. Although this is not always true, it's always the best assumption with your children, and if you are going to err, err in this direction. Even when you're wrong, your positive expectations and assumptions will encourage your child to perform according to them. If you're going to have self-fulfilling prophecies, this is the right type to have. In addition, the positive spin-off of cutting others some slack is that there is less stress on you. If you assume that your children want to do the right thing, then when they don't, you will find it easier to help them find ways to do the right thing. This is a variant of the "golden rule"—think of others as you would have them think of you.

Time to Be Alone to Relax and Think

Sometimes we get so busy that we don't have time to regroup, survey the broad landscape of our lives, and put things in perspective. This takes some time to do and, in today's busy world, doesn't come easily. A regular walk in a quiet spot, an exercise period, or a meditation or prayer period is what is needed. Whatever your beliefs, this is an important part of a balanced life and a composed mind. If you have a spouse, depend on him or her to be with the kids during this time. If not, get a sitter, or exchange time to watch your friend's kid in return for your watching her kids.

The Ability to Treasure Times of Relative Happiness

As they say, "Take time to smell the roses." Don't expect times of happiness to last, but do expect them to return. Be sure to notice when your child has a relatively better day and be thankful for it. Praise your child for it. Ponder on it and take pride and pleasure in it. Enjoy other aspects of life that are too easily overlooked: a beautiful sunrise or sunset, a gentle rain, a good grade on your child's homework. Keeping a focus on the positive encourages more positive times to emerge in the future and subtly but surely shapes your child's behavior and the behavior of others around you.

Taking Charge: How to Get What You Need from Your Personal Life

Get a Hobby

If you don't already have one, get one. If you have had one, get started again and keep it going. It's often better if this is something you do with others, as the commitment to do it with others will often help you keep on track. Some hobbies are easier than others, in that they take less time, are less expensive, or do not demand that you get someone to watch the kids. But regardless, pick something you like, and stick with it. It's not selfish: It's in the interests of your family and everyone else's well-being as well. Happier parents make happier families.

Diet and Exercise

This is a hard area for all of us. Regularly fitting this into my routine is often tough. For example, my exercise of choice is jogging. But what I have found is that I must have a running partner if I am going to stay with it and be regular. It is a lot easier to be consistent if I have committed to a friend or neighbor to show up for a brief run than if I just try to force myself out of bed and no one else is waiting for me. The same thing is true for dieting. I tend to tell others about my diets and then do it with them. I may set a goal to lose some weight, but I am not alone: Usually either a friend or a family member has set a similar goal, and we then get to provide each other support and encouragement.

Reward Yourself

I reward myself, just like I do for my kids: I keep a chart on the refrigerator, where I post my goals and rewards. Whether my latest goal happens to involve running, losing weight, or coming home from work on time, I set up a chart for all to see. This allows my spouse and kids to encourage me when I keep my own goals and needle me when I don't. And the public commitment ensures that I don't cut corners, and that everyone else knows what I want to do.

Give Yourself an Allowance

Budget an allowance for yourself. Spend at least as much money on yourself as on your spouse or child. This is hard for some parents: In their minds, kids always come first. This is nonsense. If kids always come first, how do they learn to respect other adults, to be polite, to take others' needs into account? So you must model self-care and self-caring if you want your children to like themselves and respect themselves as adults. Water rises no higher than its source!

What to Do When Your Personal Life Leaves Something to Be Desired

For parents of kids with ADHD, it's not unusual to end up feeling put upon, as if they have no life of their own and can't remember the last time they did something just for themselves. Some parents say they feel lonely in their own home and have also lost touch with their friends, because they never go out with them anymore. Others suddenly notice they're getting sick all the time. Or they realize they're always letting their kids or spouse choose the restaurant, leisure activity, vacation site, or dinner menu. Here are a few tips for solving these personal-life deficits.

- *Unwind.* You may be on the verge of burning out. Too much, too long, basically. It's time to talk with a friend. Sometimes long periods of stress can actually change your brain's neurochemistry, making you prone to depression, excessive alcohol or drug use, or other related problems.
- *See your doctor.* Your doctor is in the position to evaluate whether the stress has actually caused a depression or other, related problem. He can also determine if you have ADHD, which will make all these tasks and demands even more challenging.
- *Are you getting sufficient time alone for yourself, really?* You may need to evaluate your R&R (rest and relaxation) opportunities. Are the burdens being shared with your spouse? Can your parents or in-laws help out? Are you keeping your hobbies up? Is it time to go on strike?
- *Revisit the quality of your relationships.* Relationships are key to mental health

---

Is *Your* ADHD Getting in the Way of Your Managing
Your Child's ADHD?: Ask Yourself These Questions

- If you have ADHD yourself, do your child's symptoms look normal to you, making it hard for you to recognize a problem in your child, and causing you to delay seeking help for your child? "Based on their observations while evaluating my son, the SpEd testers also concluded that he does have the hyperactivity piece, which I wasn't sure about (I can be hyper, too, so my activity level rivals my son's; therefore, I could not distinguish this as clearly)."
- If you have ADHD, is your own patience for dealing with your child stretched?
- Do you find it impossible to implement your child's behavior therapy programs because they seem so tedious or complicated?
- If your ADHD were treated, would your child do better? "As a result of my daughter's diagnosis, I was forced to take a hard look at my own background—I was tested as an adult (thirty-nine years old) and I have ADHD myself. The treatment plan developed for myself has had a positive impact on the relationships with my husband and daughters."
- Refer to *Driven to Distraction* by Ed Hallowell, MD, listed in Appendix D, for additional information and a self-assessment on whether you might also have ADHD.

---

and happiness. It is quite likely that you are not getting your needs met in this area. Go back and review an earlier part of this chapter, "Making Relationships Work for You."

    • *Back to the basics.* Reevaluate the steps and earlier principles outlined in Chapters 2 and 3.

Your Action Plan

Before leaving this chapter, refer again to your short- and intermediate-term action plans. You are likely to find that there are additional areas that need to be filled in. Have you spotted any additional family or personal needs, approaches that can be taken, or ultimate objectives? See my examples in the Intermediate-Term Action Plan on the next page, then do your own, both short-term and intermediate (see Appendix F for blanks).

INTERMEDIATE-TERM ACTION PLAN

Your child's needs	Approaches How will the need(s) be addressed? Resources?	Who will do it? Who else will assist and be on your child's team?	When? What is the time frame for accomplishing specific tasks?	Outcomes Intermediate-term goals and objectives
<u>Social-emotional needs</u>				
<u>Medical needs</u>				
<u>Educational needs</u>				
<u>Parent-family needs</u>				
Better marriage relationship	*Discuss with husband, consider marriage retreat or counseling*	*Both of us*	*Next Saturday evening after dinner*	
Vacation time away to recuperate	*Switch out watching my friend's child for one week, so we both can take a break*	*Who else but me does anything around here?*	*Tomorrow, when I see her*	
Less criticism from my family	*1. Write frank letter (Duh!) to my mother expressing my need for her support* *2. Give her material to read, ask her to attend CHADD meeting or doctors visit*		*When I work up my courage—talk with my friend first*	

Eight

GETTING THE BEST FROM ALL THE REST

"This has been the most painful area for me personally. We rarely get invited to any informal extended family get-togethers. I sit here typing on Easter morning because we were not included in an Easter breakfast sponsored by one of my siblings to which everyone else, including my parents, was invited. Plans are made and not shared with us, but I usually find out about them anyway."

"My family is very formal and politically correct in the way that they relate to one another. But my home can be loud, chaotic, and challenging at times, and my extended family is uncomfortable dealing with that and my son, and anything else that is unpredictable. I often feel judged and isolated. Our neighbors also have generally shunned my son, who has alienated agemates on the street with his bossy behavior. They stay away from me, too, but in a way I'm relieved, because I get so tired of making excuses for his behavior."

"I found my family to be absent— 'sorry to hear . . . let me know if I can help . . .' but then when I needed respite, they were never around. We don't get invited out much. I am not sure if it is fear of my children's behavior or not—no one will tell you that directly—but I suspect that is a part of it."

"I am currently divorced. I fear it will be difficult for me to establish a new relationship—because my son is quite challenging. If he is challenging for me, how will he be seen by others? It is a lot to ask of someone who has no kids or, even worse, has normal kids."

"I wonder, almost daily, how I'll ever manage a career while trying to raise two kids with ADHD."

Your child's mental healthcare, education, and home life are undoubtedly your top priorities, and managing these areas of life for a child with ADHD can easily take up all of your time. But your child will spend a lot of time outside the home and school, and this is where some of the thorniest problems occur. In this chapter, we

199

tackle your child's friendships and social life; extracurricular activities, such as hobbies and sports; outings, such as shopping and religious worship; and relationships with relatives. We'll also take a brief look at how you can mesh all your child- and family-related responsibilties with your career. It can be heartbreaking to watch a beloved son or daughter rejected by peers or to know that your whole family is being left out of holiday gatherings of relatives. But many parents find that as their child gets the best treatment available, begins to succeed at school, and learns methods to control his behavior at home, his new skills transfer to social settings. And there, in turn, his talents and abilities grow, and Mom and Dad get to watch him take pride in being able to mingle smoothly in the wider world.

All of the areas discussed in this chapter are thought to contribute to children's sense of self-worth or self-esteem. A good sense of self-esteem—an inner feeling of liking oneself—doesn't happen all at once, and no single factor is likely to make or break it. Nor is self-esteem an "either you got it or you don't" kind of personal characteristic. Instead, it is gradually built from your child's experiences, bit by bit and day by day. If all experiences are bad, a child learns to expect only bad things in the future, never to expect success, and to feel like she is just not good at anything. The key experiences that contribute to self-esteem are a child's peer relationships, her skills, abilities, and hobbies, and her relationships with adults. Let's consider each of these areas.

Making Your Child's Friends and Relationships Work for You

So, what can you reasonably hope for your child in terms of peers and peer relationships? Can your child make and keep friends, and what can you do to make it possible? How do you handle situations such as when your child does not get invitations to birthday parties? Or is never asked to play after school or on the weekend? Or to come to a sleepover? Or is always the one not picked to be on a team? How will your child fare in the teenage years, when dating and other peer relationships seem to carry so much weight? Can he have a "social life"? And what do you do when other adults, such as parents of your child's classmates, tell you, "I'm sorry, but your child can't play at our house anymore—he's too disruptive"?

What to Expect from Your Child's Social Relationships

At Least One or Two Friends

First, let's establish what's important. In terms of longer term healthy development and good outcomes, it is not important that your child be popular per se. Rather, it is important that he have *some* friends. It doesn't have to be many, and in fact, even having one "best friend" whom you like and who likes you may be the most essential aspect of peer relationships. What research has taught us is that the child who is *explicitly rejected* by her peers is most at risk for later problems. In fact, as best we can tell, there is very little difference in terms of outcomes between being very popular and simply being liked by a few kids. But there is a *big difference* between being liked by only one or two kids and being actively rejected by all kids. So what can you do to encourage your child to make and keep some friends? Yes, it is true that you can't make friends for your child. But there is a lot you can do to encourage friendships and make them more possible.

Fostering a Hobby, Talent, or Skill

Fostering a skill or talent in a child with ADHD can be challenging, because children with ADHD may be more likely to get frustrated at their inability to perform at a given activity, and they resist the very practice they need to get better. But sticking with this is important for a couple of reasons. First, if your child is struggling just to get by in school, she is going to feel pretty bad about herself. She is going to need some areas of strength to offset these negative feelings. Second, being good at something outside of schoolwork is an effective conduit to friendships, or at least practice with social interaction. After all, many kids' hobbies or talents are pursued in groups, whether it's a sports team, a baseball card trading club, or a children's choir.

Every child has areas of relative strength or talent. Children don't have to be superstars; they just have to feel like they can be "pretty good." Pretty good is relative; it's more in the eye of the beholder, and in this case it's your child's eye that counts. You or others may give the child some positive feedback about how she has done something, and if that area has also sparked your child's interest, your job is to kindle that spark. If your child feels encouraged and gets some satisfaction from what she has done and how she has done it, feed that germ. As one woman put it, "My advice is to carefully guard your child's self-esteem. Find something he succeeds at or enjoys that is outside of the school setting. What saved my child was his athletic ability. He was sought after for baseball and football."

Finding a skill or talent can take time, and you shouldn't be discouraged if your child doesn't hit on something right away. In the case of my own son with ADHD, it didn't really begin to happen until his high school years, when he began to experience a sense of his athletic ability. Before that time, there were a lot of frustrating moments, both for him and for us as parents. Looking back on it, I think that the most important thing we did was to remain encouraging and supportive, buoying him up when he was discouraged and wanted to quit, trying to prevent any out-and-out disasters as best we could.

If you're like me, you may find it difficult to play this role, and maybe you can learn from my mistakes: When teaching my son how to catch a baseball and, later, to hit the ball, I would get too wrapped up in the teaching role, rather than taking the time to deal with his frustration. So my son would refuse my advice on how to catch the ball, insisting instead on doing it his own way, even when it didn't work and made him even more frustrated. In response, I usually wasn't patient enough to back off from teaching him the "right way" to do it. What I needed to do instead was to support him in dealing with his frustration that the way he wanted to do it wasn't working, and then help him find a solution to his problem.

Some Happy Times

All children need some happy experiences. This is tricky, however, because happy times never last, nor should you hope or expect them to for your child. It wouldn't be the best preparation for life, would it? But they do need a reservoir of happy experiences that they can draw on to create hope and sufficient optimism to face the future and approach life with confidence that good things can and will happen. In any given day, you can expect your child to have a whole variety of moods, from anger and frustration, from sadness and disappointment, to pleasure, even to joy. If nothing in life is giving your child some satisfaction and pleasure, then it is time to reevaluate his needs and see if a different approach or intervention is needed. A child who is never happy may be demoralized, or even clinically depressed, and may need a specific intervention for depression (see Appendix G).

Don't make the mistake of thinking you're responsible for creating happy experiences for your child. Just like developing friends, you cannot make this happen. All you can do is set an appropriate stage for the players to do their parts. But if the play is a disaster, as children's events and experiences sometimes are, you will want to be there to help your child pick up the pieces—by being understanding, commiserating with him, helping him feel better, and trying perhaps to anticipate and plan for better experiences next time. Your patience, your support and understanding, and your reinforcement of his or her own strengths will see most kids with ADHD through to a successful outcome.

Other Adults

You have a lot to do in helping your youngster given the need to balance all of the elements of home, family, homework, school, healthcare, and basic parenting. In spite of all you do, most children will still need other adults they really like to be with. So unfair as it seems, at times she will feel that you "have to" love and like her, and because you are the parent, it "doesn't count" in the same way. One or more other adults that your child likes being with and who communicate a sense of fun and enjoyment in return to your child can be really good for her self-esteem. This might be an uncle or aunt, a coach, a grandparent, or a friend of the family. It might even be a volunteer from your church or a youth club, a scoutmaster, or someone from a Big Brothers (Big Sisters) organization. For parents who are separated or divorced, the involvement of the other parent in the child's life can be very important. Even if the two parents no longer have a good relationship, support for each other's role with the child is a key component in children's longer term adjustment. Regardless of who fills this role, having some extra adults to spend time with your child has some benefits for you, too. When your child is with someone else, you both get a break from each other! You should try the Big Brothers (Sisters) organizations in your area (see *www.bbbs.org*), as well as the State/Local Resource Directory for Children With Disabilities website for other support services closest to you (*childrenwithdisabilities.ncjrs.org/states.html*).

Taking Charge of Your Child's Social Life

Getting What Is Needed for Your Child's Friendships and Relationships

Even though you cannot predict or control how your child's friendships and peer relationships will unfold, there are several things you can do to maximize the likelihood of success or, when things go wrong, to limit the damage. For one parent, the key was simply constant exposure to other kids: "I surround my son with friends and try to keep him as busy as possible. In the past, my son was really shy and scared. I've encouraged him to join in and be a part of whatever interests him. This has really boosted his self-esteem. As he sees success he is more willing to join in and try things. It is real easy for him to want to become a hermit. But I don't let him." Here are a few other ideas.

- *Schedule regular play times with a friend.* One simple thing you can do is to set up regular play times where your child might be able to invite someone over. Consistency, as in household routines (see Chapter 7) is valuable to a child's social life. Younger children, or those who have been burned by previous bad experiences, may not be able to ask another child to come over to your home. You may have to do it. You might first find out from your child about children he sees in class, or sits next to, or who is in his reading group. In the case of younger children, it might be one of the parents you happen to meet as you pick up your child at day care or after school. Striking up a conversation and finding a parent that you like with a child of similar age may a good place to begin.
- *Find a good match.* Sometimes it can be hard to find a child who fits in well with your child, because some children with ADHD have difficulties reading and responding to the social cues that are a part of normal peer relationships. This can lead others to tease your child or may make them be less likely to befriend your child. However, parents sometimes find that children with ADHD can more easily strike up a relationship with another child with similar difficulties, perhaps in part because both children are not keyed to the same social cues to which their agemates are sensitive. You may worry that your child needs to be with other healthy children with good social skills. True, but only to the extent that such interactions are not negative. Better to hang out with kids with whom they get along (as long as these children are not delinquent!), even if these kids have their own challenges, than to try to hang out with "popular" children, only to be ridiculed and rejected. At any rate, as the parent, you may have to "audition" various children to see how they get along with your child and whether a friendship might be nurtured.
- *Create structured play times and friendship opportunities.* When setting up a play time with a potential friend, rather than just turning the kids loose to fend for themselves and hoping something good happens, it may better to provide some structure for the activity: For example, you may want to take the kids to the park, to a movie, or to an ice cream or video parlor. Or perhaps you might provide an opportunity for them to play some video games on the home system, along with a batch of popcorn. Regardless, if your child has problems relating to others, either because of social awkwardness, aggression, or difficulties with taking turns, some gentle supervision

on your part may be necessary. The successful outcome of the activity might be further ensured if you, knowing your child's challenges, provide some guidance prior to the activity, possibly even setting up a simple reward system for his appropriate behavior (such as sharing, or not raising his voice) during the play period. An activity is successful even if the children can just be together without fighting and both seem to enjoy themselves. Nothing magic has to happen; just being together in a jointly enjoyed activity is sufficient for a positive impact on your child.

• *Limit the length of play times.* Children often get tired, and as with adults, tempers get short, impulse control lessens, and they may say or do things they might not do when functioning optimally. The solution? You might lessen the likelihood that your child's patience or temper will wear thin by keeping play periods relatively brief. While this strategy may apply to any child, particularly younger ones, it may be especially needed for the child with ADHD. And as your child experiences some successes with shorter play periods, you might gradually lengthen the periods of play.

Getting What Is Needed for Your Child's Skills, Abilities, and Hobbies

To develop your child's talents and abilities, most likely you are going to need some help; fortunately, a lot of help is usually available across a number of fronts. What can you do to maximize your child's chance to develop her talents and skills?

• *Expose your child to a range of activities.* You will never know whether your child might have some hidden talent or skill until she gets a chance to try it out. So early on, particularly in grade school and middle school, give your child chances to explore areas where she might develop a hobby or skill. The area may catch you off guard: My son eventually got into a sport that I never heard of, called "ultimate Frisbee," essentially a game where one passes a Frisbee up and down the field, moving it across the opponent's goal line by a series of passes to teammates. It might not even be a formal hobby per se, but might be an area of interest, such as animals. My son loved animals. Not just any animals, mind you, but things like snakes, tarantulas, and so forth. So we tried to take advantage of this interest, giving him chances to speak to park rangers and naturalists, getting him exposure to animals at zoos, and so forth. Eventually he got a snake—not my wife's favorite house pet, mind you, but my son loved it. Feeding the snake was quite an adventure, since it often entailed buying little baby mice that the snake would swallow, much to my son's fascination. It didn't go over so well with my wife when the snake escaped its cage and disappeared somewhere in the house. We never did figure out what happened.

At any rate, enrolling your child in an extramural class at the YMCA or YWCA, at your local recreation and parks department, or at your child's school may be an important part of his growing-up and learning experiences. Early on, you may want to provide more variety, gradually settling in on those areas that he enjoys most.

"I got my kids involved with martial arts," said one mother. "It is very structured and it helps boost their morale and self-esteem. It also provides activity, and self discipline that my ADHD son needed in his life."

- *Avoid overprogramming your child.* While it is a good idea to give your child a chance to try out various activities, don't knock yourself out, and don't "over-program" your child. Parents sometimes make the mistake of trying to pack too much into their child's life. On top of the challenges of schoolwork, it is a lot to ask of a child to participate in more than one, or at maximum two, additional activities. Follow your child's lead in this: If he is often tired and frustrated or resists a given activity after a couple of weeks or months of exposure, the hassle may not be worth it. Don't worry, it won't hurt anything if you decide that you have inadvertently packed too much into your child's life; you've got a long time left to raise your child. There's no sense sprinting when you need to learn to be a long-distance runner. Watch your pace. Apart from snakes and other such critters, my son didn't really get into other hobbies and areas of interest until he was in the last year of high school and early college.

- *Find other helping adults.* You can't do it all alone, because there are way too many areas for you to know about. Instead, here you will often need a teacher, coach, or tutor with exceptional patience. Also important is that person's ability to convey genuine warmth and affection to your child, so that he'll want to learn from that person. So for our son, we always tried to see that he had a helpful baseball or basketball coach, one who didn't get frustrated as easily as I did, and whom my son didn't feel he needed to challenge as much. My son also formed good relationships with other adults from our church, including some who shared his interest in animals and the outdoors, including activities such as fishing. This paid off quite well: although my son had great difficulties sustaining attention in many school-related activities, he could and would remain fixed by a fishing hole for long periods of time and prided himself on his knowledge and ability in this area. Weekends fishing often provided him a much needed chance to unwind from stressful school days, not only in high school but also in his early years of college.

If no helping adults are available to you, you may want to consider joining a church or social group that has volunteer adults, such as Big Brothers or Big Sisters programs. If you form relationships with other parents of children with ADHD, then you may find it possible to ask someone there to spend some time with your child, and you can trade some of your time with their child in return.

- *Give the child chances to practice and develop skill.* As my son was struggling to feel good about his athletic ability during elementary and middle school, basketball camp each summer was important, since that was the place he could hone his skills, so that when the intramural basketball season rolled around, he had something to show other kids that he could do, even if he wasn't as good as those who were picked for first string on the various intramural teams. The bottom line was that we needed to find the way to help him feel that he could be a pretty good baseball and basketball player, which ended up being the case. This sense of confidence continues with him now and has led him to continue to set various goals for himself in track and other sports. Through his perseverance, he has become a darn good athlete and is recognized as such among his college peers. His "Ultimate Frisbee" team is one of the best, and he is among the best players on the team.

- *Encourage the child to pursue what interests him.* I don't have to tell you that

ADHD makes it difficult for kids to stick with tasks. But it's the ones they find boring that they have such a hard time staying with. If your child develops an interest in something, no matter how offbeat it may seem, let him run with it. "Cody, age 10," his mother proudly relates, "built a dogsled from wood in the backyard, hand-crocheted traces for the dogs, lined up neighbors' dogs to be his team, and designed two alternate routes through the neighborhood for an Iditarod. Then waited for it to snow. This was just one of his marvelous creative projects that engaged him for weeks."

What to Do When Your Child's Social Life Is Troubled

So what do you do when no one wants to be friends with your child? How about when your child refuses any hobbies? Or when he drags his feet in participating, so it just ends up being a big hassle for everyone? How about when your child and another child have just not been getting along? Or when your child has been bullied by another? (If the bullying is taking place in school, you should expect help from the faculty and administration; see Chapter 6.) Here, there are no hard and fast rules, but the following strategies may prove useful:

• Look to other parents whose children have similar difficulties. Others parent with children with ADHD are experiencing the same problems as you are. They, like you, will be eager to find chances for their child to form positive relationships with another child like yours. They, like you, want to be as supportive as they can of their child, and they, like you, hope that the parents of the other child will be just as supportive. You have a lot in common. You can find such parents through CHADD or other similar organizations; see Appendix B. Not only will these parents be more likely to be supportive of your child's need, but their child may also be less likely to rely on social cues that sometimes cause children with ADHD to be rejected by others.

• Finding a good friendship match can take a while. Don't be overly distressed. Keep looking and be patient. This can take a while, and your child's self-esteem or future won't be destroyed by struggles in this area. Having one or more friends *in the long run* is what is important, not a friend this day, this week, or this month. Of all the ADHD children I have worked with, I have never met one who didn't eventually form some constructive friendships.

• If your child is giving you a hard time and resists any new activities, remember the broken record technique: Simply repeat to your child, while not losing your cool: "I know you don't want to do this, but it is important for you to try new things. We'll try it for a couple of months, and we'll see how it goes." Another good strategy might be to let your child pick one of several activities: Don't say, "Would you like to do _____?" Never ask a yes–no question if you are not willing to accept a no. Instead, say, "We're going to let you choose one of the following things to do: what would you prefer, *x*, *y*, or *z*? It's your choice."

• Talk with other parents with a child with ADHD. What has worked for them? Often there are a host of good ideas that other parents have developed and found to work for them and their child. Although I have tried to identify lots of them in this book, I'll never cover them all. Ask other parents who have been there, seen it, and done it!

• Get to know the neighborhood parents whose children are potential friends for your child. For example, if there are events such as neighborhood parties, swim teams, or other such activities, look for chances to get to know those parents. Perhaps you can invite another family with a child who might be a potential friend over for an afternoon barbeque? Or is there an opportunity for you to host a social event for parents of neighborhood kids, perhaps a "back-to-school" social event for parents who have children the same age as yours?

• Sometimes you need a bit of "honey" to sweeten the pot and to get your child to try out new things. This may be done by a simple behavioral or reward program that you can set up on your own. See Chapter 5 and Appendix I if you need a refresher on how to do this. Or if the resistance your child is showing is fairly pervasive and encompasses many more areas than just her unwillingness to try out new activities, have you sought professional assistance in behavioral therapy? Consult your child's doctor or other experienced parents as to who is expert in behavioral treatment in your areas.

• Avoid saying "Your child said . . ." and instead say, "One of my concerns about my son is that he's having such a hard time making friends" to lead gently into recruiting the other parents' help.

• Reevaluate. Could your child be depressed? Are the problems greater than his simply refusing activities or not having friends? Or could you be too impatient?

EXERCISE 1

How to Respond When Your Child Says No One Likes Him or Her, That He or She Doesn't Get Invited to Things, and Feels Bad.

Try this dialogue on for size. Then make up a new one of your own.

YOUR CHILD: I hate school, and I don't want to go. I don't have any friends, and kids are mean to me.

YOU: [Whatever the problem, *always* respond first by listening, repeating back to make sure you understand before attempting to reassure; you need to know what has happened to set off these feelings.] It sounds like you're feeling very bad about school. Things didn't go very well today, and you feel bad about it?

YOUR CHILD: Bobbie is having a birthday party and inviting other kids, but said he won't invite me. He called me a "doofus"; then the other kids laughed.

YOU: I'm so sorry. [Big hug!] You are definitely not a "doofus." That must have made you feel so bad.

YOUR CHILD: I hate Bobbie.

YOU: I know how you must feel. I guess that sometimes kids do mean things, and they don't stop to think how it makes others feel. Part of growing up is learning how to respectful of others, and sometimes kids make mistakes. Bobbie made a mistake. Hopefully as he gets older, he'll learn not to be mean to others.

YOUR CHILD: It's not fair that I can't I go to the party.

YOU: Sounds like the party wouldn't be so much fun if he hasn't learned not to be mean. Maybe he's not such a good friend? No one can be friends with everyone.

YOUR CHILD: Yeah, he's mean.

YOU: It's important that everyone find out who their friends are. And maybe you and Bobbie don't have to be good friends, even though it's important to be polite and not mean. But sometimes it takes a while to figure out who your friends will be. How about we invite Clark over on Saturday, and you both can have a special trip to the video parlor and ice-cream store? It'll be your own party, and you can see if maybe you and Clark can be friends?

YOUR CHILD: OK.

Resources to Help Kids with ADHD Socialize

You have a range of options that may work for you, if you are especially concerned about your child's socialization abilities. These vary from region to region, so what works for one parent may not work for another. Start by asking other parents on CHADD Chat (*www.chadd.org*). Then also consider these options: Many organizations sponsor social occasions for kids with special needs. Check with your local school district, your closest CHADD chapter, and local units of national groups such as the Boy Scouts, Girl Scouts, 4H, and so on.

Good hobbies for kids who have a hard time sitting still and sticking with something include sports, outdoor activities with animals (4H), hiking, biking, fishing, and hunting, cheerleading, karate. Also consider anything in which your child shows a special interest. Then, hook him up with other children with the same hobby or interest.

More typical activities can sometimes be adapted so that they work for these kids.

How to Make Outings and Extracurricular Activities a Pleasure, Not a Pain

You can always steer your child toward a hobby or help him cultivate a talent. But making it possible for a child with ADHD to participate in (and be truly welcome by) an organized activity like a club or team can be really difficult. Just as the structure and routines of a school day are crafted to serve a group of children, these after-school programs rarely have the luxury of being able to attend to one individual's special needs. And because they are not mandatory the way school is, you can find your child excluded pretty readily. Fortunately, there are ways to make sure your child with ADHD doesn't miss out on this important part of childhood.

Nor should your child be barred from shopping trips, your place of worship, or dinners out. I'll tell you how parents have learned to handle these tricky situations, too.

What You Should Expect from Your Child's Extracurricular Activities

A Chance to Participate and Not Be Excluded

You may have to shop around a bit. For example, if the coach of your child's team is not understanding enough about your child's ADHD, you may need to find another team. For our son, we found some coaches to be better than others: Some seemed bound by the principal of fairness (i.e., every child should get a chance to play), while other coaches seemed more attuned to "win at all costs," even if it meant leaving some kids on the bench the whole time. This may be another chance for you to think about making sure your child gets some extra lessons, coaching, or practice, but regardless, make sure the coaching staff is understanding and supportive of your child.

Satisfaction and Enjoyment

If after a period of time the extracurricular activity seems more trouble than it is worth—your child does not seem to be enjoying it and more often than not complains about the experience, it is time to reevaluate. Is this really the activity for him? With our own son, in some instances, the activity ended up frustrating him so significantly that we pointed this out to him, noting that it might mean that we should stop the activity, since it appeared to be causing him such grief. In our case, he indicated that he wanted to continue, but he found a way to rein in his frustration, making it apparently more enjoyable (at least for us, his parents).

Growing Competence and Skill in an Area

Last, if your child hangs in there, you (and she) should have every reason to expect that she will grow better in the area. Sometimes the child may have picked the wrong area, or at least an area where her talents are limited: Our son, though short for most of his growing-up years, insisted that he wanted to become an "NBA basketball star." He kept at it, in particular practicing jumping, so he could touch the hoop. And indeed, he got better and better. Repeatedly he tried out for the junior high and high school basketball teams, never quite making the grade. The last time he tried out, in his junior year, he *almost* made it, passing through several cuts until the very end. We were so proud! Interestingly, he eventually gave up basketball, taking up running and Ultimate Frisbee. But he never gave up working on his vertical jump, and he now can grab the top of the hoop with both hands. He's still working on it, with the goal of eventually "stuffing it."

What to Expect from Outings with Your Child

Making outings work is challenging. What you can expect will really depend on your child's age, how well his symptoms are controlled, the nature of the outing, and the level of adult support and supervision. Don't leave home without it. For example, a trip to the library might be a disaster, since it is not particularly interesting, and a child might become easily bored. But if he loves animals, a trip to the zoo might be terrific . . . if he doesn't wander off and get lost. So the long and short of it is, these activities have to be thought through carefully, based on what your really know about your child, his interests, strengths, the outing itself, and so forth. Don't get in over your head too quickly, as this parent experienced: "I found early on that it was too difficult to go out in public with my kids. I was physically and emotionally exhausted after one store. I started planning all of my activities for when the kids were not with me (in school, at their Dad's, etc.)."

Taking Charge of Your Child's Extracurricular Activities and Other Outings

• For sports or hobbies with adult supervision, don't settle for just any team or coach. You may want to ask adults running extracurricular activities what their philosophy, strategies, and so forth, are for dealing with kids. Select them just as carefully as you would a teacher. If you are worried or uncertain, you may want to discuss your child's difficulties with a prospective coach ahead of time. If he or she is sympathetic and/or has had experience dealing with children with ADHD, you may have the right person. Leave him a brochure to educate him, and gauge his response in a follow-up conversation. In the same way, know the adults who are leading an outing. How supportive and understanding are they? Can you prepare them, as you might a coach?

• Try to expose your child briefly to a range of settings before settling into one direction or another.

• Volunteer to serve on the team, activity, or outing. Be an assistant coach or field trip parent monitor. Sometimes this is the best way to ensure that other adults both learn about and are responsive to the special needs of children with ADHD. In effect, be part of the solution, not part of the problem; find strategies that will help others (such as the coach, who has a lot to do), as well as help you get your child's needs met. This works well, in my observation, the younger the kid is. You can be there to intervene and remove the kid if he misbehaves, before the problem makes it impossible for him to continue to participate. And you can help manage and encourage the child and even educate the other kids about ADHD and how to deal with it. But when kids get older, you may need to go back to the first strategy (don't settle for just any team or coach), or identify behavioral goals for you child in that setting, and make them a part of your overall behavior program. Be careful, however. Don't set too many behavioral programming items in place, or you will overwhelm yourself and the child. Which are the most important two or three to tackle right now? You have lots of time; the others can wait.

• Remember, relationships with adults who are running extracurricular activities are key. If your child does not feel liked and appreciated by these adults, and particularly if you pick up bad vibes as well, don't push it. It's not likely to work.

• Negotiate with the school if your child doesn't qualify for team sports and other activities because of his ADHD. It's not uncommon for a child with ADHD to be good at a sport or other skill, yet most schools have academic eligibility requirements for participation in extracurricular athletics. All too often, a child who is in demand for his skills in basketball or football will find himself excluded from the team because he doesn't have the required grades. If the school won't negotiate, try a city or county league or team. Or a child who performs beautifully in an extracurricular area that interests her will be denied the privilege of participating because faculty or other staff will see that her behavior during class is often below par and assume that it will carry over into another setting. Of course, it's an ironic fact of ADHD that this is often not the case. Teach them this, and consider taking them a letter from your doctor indicating that the sports activity is "medically necessary" for self-esteem development.

• Should you set up a special, time-limited behavior management programs that work at home and in school for trips away from home?

What to Do When Extracurricular Activities or Outings Don't Work for Your Child

So what do you do when your child is unwelcome in all the available organized activities nearby? Or if your child doesn't want to play or participate because no one likes him, or because he's "no good"? Or if the coach of the team/extracurricular activity doesn't feel able to "handle" your child?

• Find a summer camp program. A concentrated period of activity or practice in a given skill can be very helpful. Nowadays there are art camps, basketball camps, computer camps, even ADHD camps; you name it, it's out there. Let the buyer beware, however. Not all camp programs may be sufficiently supportive to provide a good experience for a child with ADHD. Find out what other parents have done. Go to CHADD Chat (*www.chadd.org*) and get advice.

• Talk with other parents about which experiences are best and most supportive of children with ADHD and related special needs.

• Organize your own activity or outing, joining with parents of other children with ADHD or special needs. Or check with local CHADD chapter members or State/Local Resource Directory for Children With Disabilities to find out about other possible resources in your area (*childrenwithdisabilities.ncjrs.org/states.html*).

Making Extended Family and Friends Work for You

It would be great if extended and friends were as fully supportive as we'd like, but this may be the exception, rather than the rule. In many parents' experience, grandparents, aunts, uncles, and friends may not understand what you're dealing with: "As far as my parents go, they are truly a different generation—explain as you may, they are sympathetic but not able to grasp the meaning of what ADHD truly entails. It's better between me and my siblings—we educate one another. We read books on bipolar disorder and ADHD. We try to look at each other and say, 'OK, he's having a moment!' " You may not be able to expect the same from friends, however: "Sadly, we've lost friendships because of ADHD. But we've clung to those who try to understand and lend support." So what *do* you have the right to expect from those outside your immediate family?

What You Should Expect from Your Extended Family and Friends

Support and Empathy

Others have no right to judge you if they haven't walked in your shoes. But the simple fact is, even those we know best may not get it. There are a lot of misconceptions out there, and sadly, our loved ones are just as prone to them as strangers are. If we have time and energy to spare, we can hope to educate them. One parent, who said that some of her family members and friends "tend to think I'm taking the 'easy way out' with regard to medicating my son," made it her "personal mission" to educate others

> "so that they are made very aware of how knowledgeable we are on the matter and going with the most current medical information available, to give our son the best possible chance at a healthy, productive and fruitful life. I've learned to disregard most opinions and have come to rely on a few tried-and-true friends that now better understand ADHD. Honestly, I sort of understand, because my perception was always that ADHD wasn't real. Until I had a child diagnosed, medicated him to help him cope, and had seen the differences, I always internally judged parents who would 'claim' to have a child with ADD or ADHD."

Not everyone is willing to add educating others to their already lengthy list of responsibilities, however. After all, support and empathy are not much to ask from people who already care about you, and if they don't offer it, is educating them worth your time?

Not Judging or Blaming You for Your Child's Problems

Enough said here. As outrageous as it is when it happens, as this parent attests—"I have found that families with no knowledge of ADHD can be extremely judgmental of both bad behaviors and our decision to use medication," it is all too common. If your "friends" seem to blame or judge you vis-à-vis your child, is this a friendship that you can afford?

Advice, But Only When You Ask for It

Here's another all-too-familiar story:

> "Most of the bad advice I got (and still get) is from people who *mean* well. They assume that if I were more strict with him, I wouldn't have problems. Every day

I hear, 'If he were *my* kid . . .' Like somehow my bad parenting has resulted in his problems. When I insisted there was something bigger going on, nobody wanted to accept that. For some reason it was easier for family and friends to blame me for the problems."

You may need to be blunt here: "I appreciate your opinions, but I really think you need to get more education in this area." Relatedly, they ought not to be questioning or second-guessing your decisions. You'll have enough self-doubts and uncertainty all by yourself, without additional help.

Kindness toward Your Child

If your friends or relatives do not have a good relationship with your child, you will need to limit your child's exposure to them.

Willingness to Spend a Little One-on-One Time with Your Child

In the case of a close relative, such as an uncle, aunt, parent, or grandparent, it is not unreasonable that such persons should be willing to try to help out a little. If not, again, you may need to limit the amount of exposure of your child to that person, as well as any family demands that you allow that person to place on you: Your child is the first priority, and your obligation to other family members comes second: If they can't support you in your need to help your child, how much time can you take to assist them?

Taking Charge of Your Relationships with Extended Family and Friends

To the extent that you can, being proactive may enable friends and relatives to be more supportive to you and your child over the long run; thus, effort in these directions might be a good investment.

First, take the opportunity to provide information to your extended family and to close friends that your family sees often. This might include handouts from doctors, information about ADHD, the role of medications, behavioral strategies, parenting tips, and so forth.

Second, if you think your child's disorder will create problems or require accommodations at family gatherings, consider holding an informal family meeting to talk about how you can ensure that your child (and your family) won't be excluded from the activity, while your extended family and friends won't be put to too much trouble either.

Third, it might be useful to designate a "go to" adult family member and/or friend with whom your child feels comfortable, who can be contacted for help in emergencies or whenever you're not available.

Fourth, make your expectations clear. Ask what types of help, compromise, and accommodations your family and friends feel comfortable offering you and your child. If these accommodations don't square with your child's and family's needs, stay away from those situations.

And last, give family members and friends permission to talk to you openly about their observations and concerns. If they can ask honest and open questions, communication is enhanced, and you may have additional opportunities to educate them about ADHD and your child's needs.

What to Do When You Have Trouble with Relatives and Friends

When your child isn't welcome at holiday gatherings at others' houses, when your child's cousins and the children of close friends avoid him in public, when your own parents or other relatives try to interfere in your child's treatment, or when your extended family or friends blame you for your child's problems, try these simple strategies:

- Minimize time spent at gatherings where your family feels uncomfortable or unwelcome.
- Bring a diversion for your child to minimize disruption. This might be some activity (such as a portable Game Boy) that will engross your child sufficiently to keep her occupied.
- Take a baby-sitter along who can pay exclusive attention to your child.
- Buy a book on the disorder and encourage blaming family members or friends to read it. Mention that new information is available on the disorder that the person might not be aware of.
- When all else fails, remember that your child comes first. Those who insist on blaming you or excluding your child should be avoided. You may need to blunt, telling them to mind their own business, or whatever it takes to clarify that your child is your first priority.
- If you are up to it, a final step might be to ask a faultfinder or harsh judge where he is getting the information that leads to that conclusion, to defuse the situation. He may have a good idea; if so, you will want to learn about it.
- How about suggesting to relatives that your family be invited to family gatherings but that you be trusted to use your own judgment about arriving late and leaving early or participating in only the most important occasions?
- Don't forget the power of humor. You should try to defuse accusations and criticisms with lighthearted responses when you know that logic will not be persuasive.
- Don't take it personally. When a person proves to be resistant to logic, appeals to compassion and reason, remember that this is not about you. It is about that person's lack of understanding.
- Perhaps you need to seek out other sources of social support for your child and even your family. Another child who has a parent with similar struggles?
- Apply behavioral management strategies, with rewards and consequences for the period when you are at the family gathering.
- Prearrange use of your car or a separate bedroom in a more isolated part of the house for time-outs if such are needed. Or agree that one of two parents will

be on call, to work directly with the child, while the other parent socializes. Take turns on guard duty.

- Last but perhaps most important, in the words of one parent: "Sometimes when the people in your life can't or won't give you what you need emotionally, you have to give it to yourself or surround yourself with those who are capable of giving you that support."

Making Your Employer/Employment Work for You

Here are some approaches that families have used to "make their employer work for them":

"I quit working full time and took part-time positions so that I would have the energy to be the best mom I could be for him."

"Unfortunately, I have had to quit work for the past fourteen months in order to mange my son's ADHD. However, although money is much tighter now, we are fortunate enough to be able to do this. My contract for work was in negotiation and it was good timing for the decision. I was going to go back to work last September when school started, but I quickly realized that my son needed my extra support. Now that his special ed help is moving along, I will probably go back to work."

"I am very lucky right now that my job allows me some flexibility. I have not had to make any changes—however, I would like to change jobs, and one of the reasons I don't is fear that a new employer would *not* be as flexible and understanding."

"Both my husband and I work from home a great deal. It helps us manage this situation."

"I quit an out-of-home job to stay home and work (I was lucky enough to find some at-home jobs that I can do, so I can raise my kids and be there for them)."

"As the 'mom,' I have changed jobs to accommodate the needs of our family . . . not just the ADHD. Working full time, running a home, and being a mother of two very athletic, under-age-ten boys is challenging in itself. Adding a stressful management position, a husband that works sixty hours a week, and a child with ADHD to the mix was more than a body can bear. I now work in a less stressful position, on a part-time (twenty to twenty-five hours per week) basis from my home and everything else has fallen into place. *I've been able to* have 100 percent of something instead of fifty percent of everything, to *accommodate* my husband's work schedule, the kids' sports schedules, doctors' appointments, and down time. All in all, it was just what the doctor ordered." *(cont.)*

"I had been job hunting for a couple of years with little luck. However, I *was* offered a job that I turned down so that I could stay home. We felt that with Thomas entering middle school, and with what we recalled from our daughter's teenage years, it would be better to have a parent that could devote more attention. Our plan is to continue down this path until Jake graduates from high school. I will then reenter the paid labor force."

Your Action Plan

Once again, before leaving this chapter, refer to your short- and intermediate-term action plans. You should find that a few additional areas need to be filled in, and you likely have now gotten some new ideas about approaches to be taken and/or ultimate objectives.

Parents' Voices

"We had to give up on some family members—quit going to family dinners, and so forth, on one side of the family. It is sad. Cousins laugh at him and don't make him feel welcome. We finally got to the point that we realized that this family really wasn't worth the pain they caused all of us. We tried educating them, but they insist that he could control his behavior if he wanted to. We have friends that are more important to us than family members. We feel that it was best not to let him be intimidated by uncaring family members. (We didn't need it either!)"

"Oh, boy! Family: Our family has been supportive throughout our challenges. However, it was very easy for them to blame us (the parents) and give advice about how to best handle our son. For instance, some thought we should have been more strict. Some were in denial that ADHD even exists, and they wanted to hold our son accountable for things that were not within his control. Now that he is receiving medication, special ed support, and counseling, my family sees the difference and they are impressed. It was lack of education that prevented them from understanding."

"Friends: Unfortunately, my son gained a reputation for the four years before meds! There are families who still don't want my son over at their houses because of his impulsivity that was difficult to control. Understandably, it took too much effort for other parents to have him over. However, this year seems to be a good year. We received feedback from parents who did have my son over and they said, 'What a change! He's so delightful! We had some nice conversations and we really enjoyed having your son over.' Whew! I hope we are getting over the 'reputation factor.' "

"I have a very supportive family, although I get very tired of hearing about how I should do one thing or another to deal with my son. My daughter has always felt like the black sheep of the family—and she is. My sister's children always seem so perfect. My brother's child is in all the honor classes. Mostly what my daughter hears is how she needs to do things differently; everyone is always telling me how we should handle things. She feels like she is never good enough. People act like she is this way on purpose."

"My family is wonderful but they don't 'understand' my son at all. I don't think or expect anyone to really. The only people that truly understand my son and our situation are of course other parents of children like him. I love talking to other parents like me. It's a very lonely world when you don't have anyone to tell your concerns, fears, or experiences to that really relates to what you're saying. I listen to other parents talk about how well their child might be doing in a sport or their grades, or whatever. The conversations I have about my son are typically about how his behavior has been at school and/or home, or what modifications are we working on this week."

"His grandfather says he wishes they knew back then what they know now about this. He feels certain he had ADHD as a child. We just smile, because the entire family knows he's ADHD as an adult, too. Ethan is a very lovable but very challenging child. His father and I are divorced but continue to be the best of friends and work very hard to effectively coparent both children."

"Although most neighbors and friends are uncomfortable around him, a neighbor who works with him on small engine repair will work with him for shorter periods instead of having him hang out like he does our other son. My dad, even though he knew our son had the diagnosis, would say that he would take him for a month and 'straighten him out,' and he would argue and try to fight with him (we were told by family counselors not to leave our child alone with his grandfather). One friend advised spanking him, I withdrew from that friendship."

"The lack of support from the people we love most when we were at our lowest was the hardest thing to handle. They just don't want to take the time or energy to learn the best way to handle our son. So, as a result, we have pulled away from a lot of people and live in our own little world. They know where we are and what we are all about. If they feel like dealing with us, they are welcome anytime, but I don't go out of my way anymore to try to get them to understand

(cont.)

our situation. It is very painful, but I just rely on my resolve that I have dealt with my son the way I see fit and the way I see best."

"I got a lot of mouth from family about it being more a behavioral thing—and at times a 'you're not disciplining him' response. But as we've moved through the process, they see the difference in him and what a much more enjoyable child he is to be around since. And, to be honest, I didn't listen to them anyway! He's my baby and I knew what had to be done. My brother is a teacher and he balked at the 504 plan. I just ignored it. We're all allowed to have our own opinions!"

"Putting him on the right medication has improved his world in a million ways. He feels better, he feels more in control, he demonstrated better self-discipline, he has a much healthier relationship with his brother and his peers (socially). His father and I are divorced, but it has been hard because his father feels like he doesn't needs his meds on the weekends and he feels like he does. That has been difficult to deal with. My son also spent about three years (ages four to seven) without getting invited to one birthday party. That was devastating as a parent. He now gets invited all the time!"

"One of the things I often encounter is the 'casual remark' about ADHD made in social situations. This might be compared to a racist or sexist comment, but it is about people with ADHD, and it is made with the assumption that no one in the room has ADHD or has a child who has it. I do not let these remarks affect me emotionally. I do think it is sad, though, to think that children might have to deal with hearing these comments. A child would lack the frame of reference to understand that the person is misinformed, and he or she might come away feeling 'flawed' or 'bad.' Because of this, I try to provide correct information in a nonthreatening way whenever I hear someone make a derogatory comment about people with ADHD."

"The schools basically have given all that we've asked for. We are educated on the IDEA and 504 laws, and consider ourselves the true professionals with regard to our son's education and health. We are his number one advocates!!! Ryan is about to complete second grade and has been on A-B honor roll all year. We do employ a private reading tutor that he sees weekly, and now he is reading about a full year above grade level. We've instituted a reward system at home, and he is doing well behaviorally at school. He does experience some teasing and is very sensitive to that. Social deficits remain as our biggest hurdle. (Of importance to note: Other children that seem to have many more 'problems' than Ryan receive no services at all, because the parents haven't been proactive or, for whatever reason, opt not to pursue help.)"

"The single most important piece of advice to a new parent? You can be your child's number one advocate and the expert with regard to all facets of his or her life, but you must educate yourself, and you have to be comfortable with relying on the currently available medical and psychological information, as well as relying on your instincts and feeling good about your decisions, without second-guessing yourself all the time. Nobody else—*nobody*—can do the job for your child as well (or with the love and determination) as you can, so hop on board and enjoy the ride as best you can. Your child is worth it and with your help he can make it! Rest in that hope!"

"You need to be on the lookout for people who can lower your child's self-esteem. Children hear and see more than you think. You need to be careful when talking about your child to other people and make sure they are careful when speaking about your child to you."

Nine

LOOKING AHEAD

"My son who is in fourth grade now is finally doing well enough that he (on his own) decided to try out for the lead in the school musical. He got the part and was great; he wowed everyone (parents and kids alike). It was one of the proudest moments of my life. These kids can be amazing if they get the help they need."

"He still has a way to go at sixteen years old, and our challenges are different now with driving and girls, and being allowed out alone to make good decisions, but I have a more successful student and son now. When each little step of progress is noticed, you will be overwhelmed with the 'baby steps' and progress that your child can attain with the right treatment processes."

"We have only one child. We spend a lot of time after school helping to educate our son. We have had to do that since he was young. He is getting more mature and responsible and we are beginning to feel that he will ultimately be able to be on his own in education. We function as his coaches and it works well. It has been a very long struggle, but it's paying off and he's a great teen."

"Don't give up. . . . There is a light at the end of the tunnel. Our daughter is seventeen going on eighteen and will graduate next year from high school. She carries a 3.5 GPA and is looking forward to college. She has eleven of the fourteen criteria for hyperactivity and will have it for the rest of her life. With the help of diet, medication, counseling, and just due diligence by Mom and Dad, we have been able to get her to the point that she is almost grown."

"When you have a child facing challenges, it is the little things that you remember. It is the A on the essay, when essays used to be torture. It is the invitation from the girl to go to the prom, when social interactions come so hard. It is the meeting, previously forgotten even with weeks of nagging, remembered after the medication change; or the thank you note written without being prompted. It is my husband's 'Aha' that he really has a brilliant kid with ADHD, not a lazy one with an attitude."

One parent found the perfect words to express the uncertainty that all of us feel about our kids, ADHD or not: "As you watch a child with ADHD grow, you don't have a clue what the outcome will be. You work hard on faith. Eventually, hopefully, you come to a point where you can see what the outcome is going to be, and then you know that it is a developmental disability. Someone needs to work hard at explaining that to families, because it makes the hard early years seem worthwhile." So what does the future hold for your child with ADHD? How can you stay on track, getting the best care for your son or daughter, while taking good care of yourself and the rest of your family? Will all your efforts be worthwhile? In this chapter, I show you what other parents have accomplished by becoming effective managers of their child's care. The process is not perfect, much less easy. The outcome is not certain. But by developing and implementing your short-term plans, taking it one day at a time, and looking for and rejoicing in small victories, you will certainly begin to see results, just like these mothers and fathers have.

Challenges will still arise, and nothing can prevent true disasters occurring to any of us. That is just a part of life. But coming to terms with life and all of its challenges, including accepting the challenges of parenting a child with ADHD, can also broaden and deepen our capacity to care, to love others, to make the most of what we have (which is likely to be quite a lot), and even to accept ourselves. I am reminded of the story of the two would-be farmers, each of whom was given a plot of land. The first farmer argued against the lot he was dealt, feeling that it was unfair and that he should have been given a larger and more fertile parcel of land. The second, wiser farmer put his hand to the plow, removing rocks and stumps, building irrigation ditches, and working fertilizer into the barren land. In time, the first farmer had little to show for his efforts and anguish; the land remained untilled and barely productive. The second farmer found that the apparently barren plot of land in fact produced many remarkable fruits and crops. The major difference lay not in the land, but in what was put into it, not just in water and nutrients, but also in personal sweat and tears.

As parents, we can never know the future for our children, much less for ourselves. All of our initial hopes for our children's futures are rarely realized. But forming short-term plans, greeting successes as well as setbacks, and factoring these results into our next set of short-term plans creates a method for making good use of the cards we are dealt, and often even improving our draw in the next hand. "Chance favors the prepared mind." So as we read the following comments from real parents, we need to ask, "What were these parents given at the start? How did they handle it? What did they then put into what was given them? What have they received get in return?" Do not give in to notions that your child is like "damaged goods" or that you can't make a difference. Or that you and your child are destined for unhappy lives. These notions are *never* accurate, but believing them can make it so. Instead, take heart that many others have walked (and are walking) the same paths as you! Reach out, get help from other parents. Give help in return, and you will find that your burden and your child's burden will truly be lightened. But don't take it from me. Let's close this book by hearing it from the true experts . . . other parents who have walked in your shoes.

Parents' Voices

"Please, please, let that child know how much he is loved. The child feels every-one shunning him and feels unlovable. That is intolerable! Every day, tell your children what their unique gifts are and make an effort to get them involved in activities where they can feel competent."

"Our adoption agency assured us that our son was healthy. It was hard to un-derstand—when we had no other children—what his behaviors were all about. At first I felt that I should have never had a child—that I really was in-competent. It even crossed my mind that if I really loved this child, I should take him back to the adoption agency so that they could find a mother that could get him to comply with the simplest of rules. After we found out about ADHD, it took some time before I learned that I was a very good mother! I just had to get used to the fact that I would have to work harder and get far fewer rewards! The hardest thing was (and still is) learning to change my expecta-tions and hopes for my child. I'm a great parent—my kid is a great kid. I wanted him to have at least a college education, I wanted him to have friends, I wanted him to be happily married. None of this has happened yet (he is twenty-six). It is hard to watch him struggle, hard to see him mistreated by oth-ers, and hard to see him lose his self-confidence and enthusiasm for life. He is lonely. There always seems to be a daily crisis in his life. I'd like to see him ex-perience some peace! It is very hard for me to watch others not accept him for who he is. The good things are that he is self-sufficient. He lives on his own. He has a few friends. He has a hobby—racing cars—and he is quite good at it. And he is attending the community college—two classes each quarter."

"When my son was four, he worried about how he would reach the gas pedal when he was old enough to drive. Now my son is eighteen and he worries about how he will ever decide what he wants to be when 'he grows up!' My point is, there will always be problems, just different levels and severity."

"Our son, as well as many other kids with ADHD, is a fun-loving, bright kid. Since he's got this tremendous energy, any kind of outdoor activity is a real pleasure. Kevin is very athletic and enjoys other people. We make his life as normal as possible, and he knows that he has ADHD, but we don't make it a big deal. At the same time, we want him to be aware that if he sits on a ball at school, it's because his teachers want to ease his activity level and make him more comfortable. He accepts it pretty well and he's actually having fun. We emphasize the fact that *everybody* is different and it takes all kind of people to make a world."

"My son and I talk a lot. Constant communication with him makes all the difference in the world. Even though I am not someone who likes to talk a lot, I force myself to listen attentively to my son and give him feedback, so that he knows I am paying attention. If a period of time goes by without this connection, it inevitably shows up in my son's behavior. Because ADHD children's worlds are much more chaotic than those without ADHD, adults must be the calming factor in their lives (every day!). So despite my son's challenges due to ADHD, I see great things for his future. I know that I have to provide him with the level of support he needs now in order to help make it happen."

"Taking my son off medicine has helped tremendously, decreasing his moodiness and the difficulty dealing with him in the evenings when he's coming off the medicine. We still must deal with his hyperactivity and lack of attention span, but that is much better than the moodiness/rebellion the medicine caused. I only hope he continues to do well in school and is able to control his hyperactivity enough that we do not have to put him back on medicine. I am divorced and, when I was dating, my son's ADHD behavior made it very difficult, embarrassing at times, to date. I have now remarried, but it has been a difficult challenge for my husband (who has no children) to accept and learn to deal with my son. My husband has done remarkably well, even though things aren't perfect."

"Through the chapter meetings and National CHADD conferences I have learned so much about ADHD that I no longer think of my children as having something wrong with them. ADHD is part of what makes them. I have also made some great friends in the chapter. Often they are the only people I can speak freely to about my children, knowing that they will understand and offer their support. I have also learned to advocate for my children and in turn have taught them to advocate for themselves."

"I think the recognition and focus on our son's giftedness (vs. the issues associated with his ADHD/LD) has had the greatest impact so far on his life. It was the medication, I believe, which allowed the focus to be effective. 'The pill is not the skill,' but the medication has allowed him to learn the skills and to be appreciated by his teachers instead of their relationship being complicated by his angry outbursts. Seeing him grow has impacted my husband's view of our son and has taken substantial pressure off of both of us."

"On a really positive side, ADD family life is never boring. It isn't sane either, but I am sure as the kids get in to their twenties we will start to hear some 'tales' of some adventures we were not privy to in years past. We also have an ADHD

(cont.)

dog. *Gosh!* If he isn't the most fun. Mischievous, annoying, and full of love despite his blunders. Kind of just like my kids!"

"There is no one thing I can point out that has been a 'big Aha!' But I can say that in those quiet moments when Tucker is asleep or absorbed in something, I look at him and remember why all of the struggles and conflicts are worth it. He is a kind and affectionate child who is *so* worth knowing! I hope to help him be a wonderful adult."

Your Long-Term Action Plan

OK, I hope it's now quite clear that you don't have to give up having dreams for your child. Most of these parents are realizing their dreams—somewhat different dreams than they started with when their child first became theirs, but *beautiful* dreams nonetheless. And what is a long-term action plan other than your realizing your ultimate dreams for your child? So as a final step in creating your action plan, dare to dream once again, and write down your long-term hopes and dreams for your child (a blank is provided in Appendix F, p. 254). And seeing his or her needs fulfilled is the dream, is it not? I've put down a few dreams of my own under the "needs" column on the left side of the example on the facing page, and to get you started.

LONG-TERM ACTION PLAN

Your child's needs	Approaches	Who will do it?	When?	Outcomes
Social–emotional needs 1. Good self-esteem, though he might struggle at times 2. A nice girlfriend (not yet, but I am still hoping!) 3. Other good friends and buddies 4. Good athletic skills, and takes pride in them				
Medical needs 1. Doesn't need meds currently, but open to future possibility 2. Good temper and self-control skills 3. Advocates for his own needs when necessary				
Educational needs 1. In college 2. Likes his studies 3. Good part-time job				
Parent–family needs 1. Good parent–son relationships 2. Son and siblings get along; they even like each other!				

Author's Note In Closing

I have learned so much from writing this book, and perhaps, like you, I have learned most from reading the stories and struggles of other parents who are a lot like me and probably a lot like you. If you are willing, I would be honored to pass on any of the lessons that you have learned to future readers. So please share these stories of success and failure with me. What has worked, and what hasn't? To give you some inspiration (as if that were needed!), here are the questions, the answer to which you have heard in the parent voices throughout the pages of this book.

- What was the hardest thing for you in accepting your child's ADHD?
- What has made the biggest difference for you in learning how to handle all of the problems you and your family have had to face as a result of your child's ADHD?
- *School systems.* Did you have any particularly challenging experience in the schools pertaining to your child's ADHD? What happened? If things are better now, what did you have to do to make things change?
- *Getting good information.* What happened along the way as you were struggling to get an accurate diagnosis? What kinds of misinformation or bad advice was pushed on you? What has been the best advice you have ever received pertaining to the overall challenges of dealing with your child's ADHD?
- *The medical system.* How helpful were doctors and therapists in your child's diagnosis and treatment? What were the biggest problems you encountered? Did you ever feel blamed? Have you changed doctors or therapists, and if so, why? How many times?
- *Families and friends.* What particular problems have you had to face from family members and friends in their accepting you and your child? Did anything really make a difference and turn things around? How has your child's ADHD affected your relationship with your spouse or other children?
- *Lifestyle changes.* Have you had to make major lifestyle changes, such as moving to find good care or schools for your child, changing jobs, quitting work, and so forth, in order to manage your child's ADHD? What happened?
- If you could give a single point of advice to a new parent with a child with ADHD, what would it be? What is it most important for them to do? What should they be on the lookout for, or be careful *not* to do?

Lastly, let me refer you to Appendix J, if you, like many parents who have been helped by other parents and mentors, want to give help to others in turn.

I look forward to hearing and learning from you. Please write to me at

c/o Making the System Work
     Peter S. Jensen, MD
     Center for Advancing Children's Mental Health
     Columbia University, Unit 78
     1051 Riverside Drive
     New York, NY 10032

APPENDICES

SAMPLE SECTION 504/ADA ACCOMMODATION PLAN

This plan lists examples of accommodations or interventions that a school district might offer a student with a disability to help him or her achieve success in school. Every student has different needs, and the plan should be customized to those needs. A profile of the needs should first be done, then prioritized. Even though some students may need more accommodations or interventions than others, it is important for parents and educators to be realistic and not try to "fix" everything at once. Choose the most critical areas of concern and then target a few accommodations or interventions that can realistically be accomplished by the team of parent, teacher, and child.

Areas of Concern

____ Activating and getting started
____ Irritability, depressed mood, sensitive to criticism
____ Memory, recall
____ Motor activity
____ Compliance
____ Academic skills
____ Sustaining attention and concentration
____ Sustaining effort
____ Impulsiveness
____ Organizing and planning
____ Socialization

Accommodations by Teacher

Physical Arrangement of Room:

____ Seating student near teacher
____ Standing near student when given directions or presenting lessons
____ Additional accommodations: _____
____ Seating student near positive role model

From Kenosha Unified School District, Kenosha, Wisconsin.

_____ Avoiding distracting stimuli (high-traffic areas, windows, heating system)
_____ Increasing the distance between the desks

Lesson Presentation:

_____ Pairing students to check work
_____ Writing key points on the board
_____ Providing peer tutoring
_____ Providing visual aids
_____ Providing peer note taker
_____ Making sure directions are understood
_____ Additional accommodations: _____
_____ Providing written outline
_____ Allowing student to tape-record lesson
_____ Having student review key points orally
_____ Teaching through multisensory modes
_____ Using computer-assisted instruction
_____ Including a variety of activities in each lesson
_____ Breaking longer presentations into shorter segments

Assignments/Worksheets:

_____ Giving extra time to complete tasks
_____ Simplifying complex directions
_____ Handing worksheets out one at a time
_____ Reducing the reading level of the assignment
_____ Allowing student to tape-record assignments/homework
_____ Providing study skills training
_____ Shortening assignments; breaking work into smaller segments
_____ Additional accommodations: _____
_____ Allowing typewritten or computer-printed assignments
_____ Using self-monitoring devices
_____ Reducing homework assignments
_____ Not grading handwriting
_____ Requiring fewer correct responses to achieve grade
_____ Providing structured routine in written form
_____ Giving frequent shorter quizzes and avoiding long tests

Test Taking:

_____ Allowing open-book exams
_____ Giving exams orally
_____ Giving take-home tests
_____ Allowing student to give test answers on tape recorder
_____ Additional accommodations: _____
_____ Giving frequent short quizzes
_____ Allowing extra time for exams

____ Reading test item to student
____ Giving more objective items (fewer essay responses)

Organization:

____ Providing peer assistance with organizational skills
____ Providing student with extra set of books for home
____ Providing student with an assignment notebook
____ Providing rules and help with getting organized
____ Additional accommodations: _____
____ Checking homework daily
____ Setting short-term goals for work completion
____ Assigning volunteer homework buddy
____ Sending daily/weekly progress reports home
____ Requesting parental help with organization
____ Supervising writing of homework assignments
____ Giving assignments one at a time

Behaviors:

____ Providing frequent, immediate, positive feedback
____ Using self-monitoring strategies
____ Contracting with student
____ Increasing the immediacy of rewards
____ Using "prudent" reprimands, avoiding lecturing
____ Using nonverbal cues to stay on task
____ Implementing a classroom behavior-management system
____ Anticipating problems and using preventative strategies
____ Additional accommodations: _____
____ Praising specific behaviors
____ Allowing legitimate opportunity to move
____ Giving extra rewards and privileges
____ Implementing time-out procedures
____ Allowing short breaks between assignments
____ Making student correct answers, not mistakes
____ Ignoring minor inappropriate behaviors
____ Supervising during transition times

Mood:

____ Providing reassurance and encouragement
____ Speaking softly in nonthreatening manner if student is nervous
____ Focusing on student's talents and accomplishments
____ Making time to talk alone with student
____ Looking for signs of stress build-up and providing encouragement or reduced workload
____ Allowing student an opportunity to "save face"

____ Additional accommodations: _____

____ Training anger control: encouraging student to walk away; using calming strategies

____ Complimenting positive behavior and work

____ Looking for opportunity for student to display leadership role in class

____ Sending positive notes home

____ Reinforcing frequently when student is frustrated

____ Using mild, consistent consequences

____ Giving student choices

Academic Skill:

____ If *reading* is weak: provide extra time, use "previewing" strategies, select text with less on the page, shorten amount of reading required, avoid oral reading

____ If *oral expression* is weak: accept all oral responses, substitute display for oral report, encourage expression of new ideas, pick topics easy for student to talk about

____ If *written language* is weak: accept nonwritten forms of reports, accept use of typewriter or tape recorder, do not assign large quantities of written work; test with multiple choice or fill-in blanks

____ If *math* is weak: allow use of calculator, use graph paper to space numbers, provide extra math time, provide immediate correction feedback and instruction by modeling the correct computational procedure, teach the steps needed to solve a particular math problem, give clues to the process needed to solve problem, encourage use of "self-talk" to problem-solve

Medication:

Physician: _____

Medication: _____ Dose: _____ Schedule: _____

Administered in school by: _____

Parent Involvement:

____ Initial assignment notebook daily/weekly

____ Provide daily consequences for bringing completed assignment notebook/progress note home

____ Call teacher(s) every _____ for feedback

____ Call homework hotline for assignments

____ Supply school with medication and necessary medical forms

____ Attend parent support group

____ Seek out parent education about ADHD

____ Seek out parent education about behavior management

____ Provide positive reinforcement for points earned in behavior program at school

____ Write questions and concerns in assignment notebook to communicate with teacher(s)

____ Community agency involvement _____

____ Break homework into smaller parts and provide frequent breaks
____ Communicate concerns to teacher(s)/counselor
____ Inform teacher(s)/counselor of medication changes
____ Get feedback from teacher(s)/counselor to give to physician at check-ups
____ Additional accommodations: _____

Special Considerations:

____ Monitor student closely on field trips
____ Inservice teacher(s) on child's handicap
____ Provide social skills group experiences
____ Develop intervention strategies for transitional periods (i.e. cafeteria, recess, assemblies)
____ Alert school bus driver
____ Provide group/individual counselor for: _____
____ Additional accommodations: _____

Participants (names and titles):

_____

_____

_____

_____

_____

_____

Sample Student Accommodation Plan: Section 504/ADA

Student: _Isa Wild_   School: _Jefferson_

Date of birth: _10/15/95_   Grade: _8_

1. Describe the nature of the concern(s):

   Isa does not return his homework assignments. Isa has difficulty with
   organization of classwork and pacing of assignments. He's easily distracted by
   extraneous stimuli, has difficulty listening to lecture and taking notes at the same time.

2. Describe the bases for the determination of disability:

   Isa was diagnosed three years ago as having attention-deficit/hyperactivity disorder.

3. Describe how the disability affects a major life activity:

   Isa's multidisciplinary team indicated that he has difficulty with daydreaming and staying
   on task at school. He is failing two classes because he has not turned in his homework.

4. Describe the services and/or accommodations that are necessary:

   Isa's teachers will provide a weekly schedule of Isa's assignments one week in advance.
   Isa will be given one copy, and one copy will be mailed to his parents. Isa will be
   seated near the front of the room in close proximity to the teacher. Isa's parents will
   provide NCR (carbonless copy) paper so that a classmate can take notes and immediately
   give Isa a copy of the notes—or the teacher will provide a copy of the lecture notes.

Review/Reassessment date: _February 3, 2004_

Participants:	Title:
Isa Wild	_Student_
Kristy Long	_English Teacher_
Jim Johnson	_Assistant Principal/504 Coordinator_
Connie Murphy	_School Counselor_
Sarah Petes	_Social Studies Teacher_
Jane Wild	_Mother_

Special Education Terms to Remember

IDEA—Individuals with Disabilities Education Act: the law that gives eligible children with disabilities the right to receive special services and assistance in school.

IEP—Individualized Education Plan: the document stating the educational program developed by a team including the parents, it specifies the exact services the individual child will receive and sets reasonable learning goals for the child.

LRE—Least Restrictive Environment: an initiative to provide children the services they need within the most natural school setting, such that the child spends as much time as possible in the general education classroom.

Related Services—those services available to the child regardless of whether he or she has been classified as a special education student. They may include physical therapy, counseling, occupational therapy, and speech/language therapy, or test modifications.

Restricted Environment—used when the LRE can't provide the necessary services or modifications. Includes special education classrooms.

Test Modifications—Extra time, additional materials, altered environments, or other changes necessary for the child to reach his/her full potential on standardized tests.

Section 504—the section of the Rehabilitation Act of 1973 that prevents discrimination against individuals with disabilities concerning program benefits and services.

PARENT/ADVOCACY ORGANIZATIONS
AND RESOURCES YOU NEED TO KNOW ABOUT

**Anxiety Disorders Association
of America**
8730 Georgia Avenue, Suite 600
Silver Spring, MD 20910
240-485-1001 (tel)
240-485-1035 (fax)
AnxDis@adaa.org (e-mail)
www.adaa.org (website)

**Attention Deficit
Disorder Association**
P.O. Box 543
Pottstown, PA 19464
484-945-2101 (tel)
610-970-7520 (fax)
www.add.org (website)

Autism Society of America
7910 Woodmont Avenue, Suite 300
Bethesda, MD 20814-3067
800-328-8476; 301-657-0881 (tel)
www.autism-society.org (website)

**Child and Adolescent
Bipolar Foundation**
1187 Wilmette Avenue
P.M.B. 331
Wilmette, IL 60091
847-256-8525 (tel)
847-920-9498 (fax)
cabf.org (website)

**Children and Adults with Attention-
Deficit/Hyperactivity Disorder**
8181 Professional Place, Suite 201
Landover, MD 20785
301-306-7070; 800-233-4050 (tel)
301-306-7090 (fax)
www.callcenter1@chadd.org (e-mail)
www.chadd.org (website)

**Depression and Bipolar
Support Alliance**
730 North Franklin Street, Suite 501
Chicago, IL 60610-7224
800-826-3632; 312-642-0049 (tel)
312-642-7243 (fax)
www.dbsalliance.org (website)

**Federation of Families for Children's
Mental Health**
1101 King Street, Suite 420
Alexandria, VA 22314
703-684-7710 (tel)
703-836-1040 (fax)
www.ffcmh.org (website)

Learning Disabilities Association of America
4156 Library Road
Pittsburgh, PA 15234-1349
888-300-6710; 412-341-1515 (tel)
412-344-0224 (fax)
vldanatl@usaor.ne (e-mail)
www.ldanatl.org (website)

National Alliance for the Mentally Ill
2107 Wilson Boulevard, Suite 300
Arlington, VA 22201
703-524-7600 (tel)
703-950-6264 (NAMI helpline)
www.NAMI.org (website)

National Mental Health Association
1021 Prince Street
Alexandria, VA 22314
703-684-7722 (tel)
703-684-5968 (fax)
www.nmha.org (website)

Parents Helping Parents: Parent-Directed Family Resource Center for Children with Special Needs
3041 Olcott Street
Santa Clara, CA 95054
408-727-5775 (tel)
408-727-0182 (fax)
info@php.com (e-mail)
www.php.com (website)

RELATED RESOURCES USEFUL FOR PARENTS AND PARENT ADVOCATES

American Academy of Child and Adolescent Psychiatry
3615 Wisconsin Avenue, NW
Washington, DC 20016
202-966-7300 (tel)
www.aacap.org (website)

AACAP is the nation's leading professional organization for child and adolescent psychiatrists. This organization provides useful information on child psychiatric providers, as well as Facts for Families—downloadable tip sheets on a variety of subjects concerning child mental health.

American Academy of Pediatrics
141 Northwest Point Boulevard
Elk Grove Village, IL 60007-1098
847-434-4000 (tel)
847-434-8000 (fax)
www.aap.org (website)

The nation's leading organization for pediatricians, the academy provides useful information on pediatric health, including ADHD, child development, and other topics of interest concerning child mental health.

Center for Mental Health Services
Division of Knowledge Development
  and Systems Change/Administration
Room 11C-16/Parklawn Building
5600 Fishers Lane
Rockville, MD 20857
301-443-1333 (tel)
301-443-3639 (fax)
www.mentalhealth.org (website)

The federal agency responsible for giving and monitoring federal block grant dollars given to states for the care of children and adults with mental disorders, CMHS also provides fact sheets for families and offers technical assistance to states in implementing new programs.

Children with Disabilities
ChildrenDisabilities@ncjrs.org (email)
www.childrenwithdisabilities.ncjrs.org
  (website)

This website is an initiative of the Co-ordinating Council on Juvenile Justice and Delinquency Prevention, which consists of nine participating Federal agencies and offices.

National Parent Teacher Association
330 North Wabash Avenue, Suite 2100
Chicago, IL 60611
312-670-6782; 800-307-4PTA (4782)
  (tel)
312-670-6783 (fax)
www.pta.org (website)

National PTA is the largest volunteer child advocacy organization in the United States. A not-for-profit association of parents, educators, students, and other citizens active in their schools and communities, PTA is a leader in reminding our nation of its obligations to children.

**National Resource Center
on AD/HD**
8181 Professional Place, Suite 150
Landover, MD 20785
800-233-4050 (tel)
www.help4adhd.org (website)

The National Resource Center on AD/HD is a program of CHADD that was established with funding from the U.S. Centers for Disease Control and Prevention to be a national clearinghouse of information and resources concerning ADHD, an important public health concern. This website is chock-full of all types of information useful to parents and families of a child with ADHD.

**Technical Assistance Alliance
for Parent Centers**
8161 Normandale Boulevard
Minneapolis, MN 55437-1044
952-838-9000 (tel); 888-248-0822 (toll-
  free number nationwide)
952-838-0199 (fax)
alliance@taalliance.org (e-mail)
www.taalliance.org/PTIs.htm (website)

Learning to advocate for their children is a critical step that all parents of children with ADHD need to take so that they can secure services for their children and ensure the success of their children in all facets of life. Funded by the U.S. Department of Education, Office of Special Education Programs, the Technical Assistance Alliance for Parent Centers establishes and coordinates parent training centers nationwide. These training centers—Parent Training and Information centers and Community Parent Resource Centers—serve families of children and young adults (from birth to age twenty-two) with disabilities. There are approximately one hundred parent centers in the United States.

Appendix C

FUNDING- AND INSURANCE-RELATED RESOURCES YOU NEED TO KNOW ABOUT

STATE-BY-STATE RESOURCES

Each state has its own insurance department to oversee all types of insurance. The following website directs you to specific sites for each state, which offer information about the local laws and how they are enforced, as well as other helpful facts for the public.

www.hiaa.org/consumer/insurance_counsel.cfm

MEDICAID WEBSITES

Medicaid is a jointly funded, federal–state health insurance program for certain low-income and needy people. It covers approximately 36 million individuals, including children, the aged, blind, and/or disabled, and people who are eligible to receive federally assisted income maintenance payments.

Within broad national guidelines that the federal government provides, each state establishes its own eligibility standards; determines the type, amount, duration, and scope of services; sets the rate of payment for services; and administers its own program. *Thus, the Medicaid program varies considerably from state to state, as well as within each state over time.*

Centers for Medicare and Medicaid Services
www.cms.gov/medicaid/default.asp

The Centers for Medicare and Medicaid Services (CMS) offers a wealth of information and a directory of state Medicaid offices on its website. It lists various resources and technical guidance such as State Medicaid Manual, Fraud and Abuse Information, and Medicaid Statistics and Data.

Ticket to Work and Medicaid Buy-in
cms.hhs.gov/twwiia

This website, another part of the Centers for Medicare and Medicaid Services (CMS), provides information on this landmark legislation, which modernizes the employment services system for people with disabilities and makes it possible for millions of Americans with disabilities to no longer have to choose between taking a job and having healthcare.

U.S. DEPARTMENT OF HEALTH AND HUMAN SERVICES

The U.S. Department of Health Human Services launched the Insure Kids Now! campaign to link the nation's 10 million uninsured children to free and low-cost health insurance. Every state has a health insurance program for infants, children, and teens whose families do not qualify for Medicaid. Many families simply don't know their children are eligible. The states have different eligibility rules, but in most states uninsured children eighteen years old and younger whose families earn up to $34,100 a year (for a family of four) are eligible.

SCHIP
www.insurekidsnow.gov/states.htm
    This website lists information for each state about health insurance for infants, children, and adolescents. Their toll-free number is 1-877-KIDS-NOW.

U.S. AGENCY FOR HEALTHCARE RESEARCH
AND QUALITY (AHRQ)

AHRQ's mission includes both translating research findings into better patient care and providing policymakers and other healthcare leaders with information needed to make critical healthcare decisions.

Choosing a Health Plan
www.ahrq.gov/consumer/hlthpln1.htm
    This website provides guidance on health plans and how to choose an appropriate one for you or your family, as well as what that plan will include.

PHARMACEUTICAL RESEARCH AND MANUFACTURERS
OF AMERICA (PHRMA)

PhRMA is the trade association for pharmaceutical and biotechnology companies. PhRMA's mission is winning advocacy for public policies that encourage the discovery of life-saving and life-enhancing new medicines for patients by pharmaceutical/biotechnology research companies.

Helping Patients
www.helpingpatients.org
    This website offers an online directory of patient assistance programs run by over forty of its member companies.

NATIONAL RESOURCE CENTER ON AD/HD

The National Resource Center on AD/HD is a program of CHADD that was established with funding from the U.S. Centers for Disease Control and Prevention to be a national clearinghouse of information and resources concerning ADHD, an important public health concern.

Public Benefits Programs

www.help4adhd.org/en/systems/public

People with mental disorders may be eligible for several forms of public assistance to meet the basic costs of living and to pay for healthcare. This website lists information on Supplemental Security Income, Social Security Disability Insurance, and Temporary Assistance to Needy Families.

GRIEVANCES

All health insurance companies have internal grievance and complaints procedures. If you have a complaint, follow the company's procedures. All states have a state health insurance commissioner. Contact that office of the state government to see what external grievance and complaint procedures may exist in your state.

A very helpful national advocacy resource is the National Health Law Program. Visit its website (*www.healthlaw.org/consumer.shtml*) to learn which states have ombudsman and consumer assistance programs and to access information on state health insurance consumer protections. This site also provides information on choosing an appropriate health insurance plan and information on which states have pharmacy assistance programs (programs that sell prescription medications at less than market price for those without or with limited insurance).

LEGAL/ADVOCACY RESOURCES YOU NEED TO KNOW ABOUT

Disability Rights

www.usdoj.gov/crt/ada/adahom1.htm

Each federal agency (including the Department of Education) has its own set of Section 504 regulations that apply to its own programs. Agencies that provide federal financial assistance also have Section 504 regulations covering entities that receive federal aid. Requirements common to these regulations include reasonable accommodation for persons with disabilities. Each agency is responsible for enforcing its own regulations. Section 504 may also be enforced through private lawsuits. It is not necessary to file a complaint with a federal agency or to receive a right-to-sue letter before going to court. For information on how to file Section 504 complaints with the appropriate agency, contact:

> **Disability Rights Section**
> Civil Rights Division
> U.S. Department of Justice
> P.O. Box 66738
> Washington, DC 20035-6738
> 800-514-0301 (voice)
> 800-514-0383 (text telephone)

Judge David L. Bazelon Center for Mental Health Law

www.bazelon.org

The Bazelon Center is an information and advocacy organization that focuses on laws, policies and regulations that affect (1) the civil rights of people with mental disabilities and, (2) access to services for adults and children with disabilities.

Legal Protection and Advocacy Strategies for People with Severe Mental Illnesses in Managed Care Systems

www.nami.org/Content/ContentGroups/Legal/NAMI_Legal_Publications.htm

This NAMI resource provides an overview of legal issues in both the public and private sectors. The manual is a blueprint for challenging decisions and practices in of-ten-complicated systems.

Your State Protection and Advocacy System
www.napas.org

To obtain legal representation, please contact the protection and advocacy sys-tem in your state. Protection and advocacy systems in each state are federally funded to assist people with mental or developmental disabilities in understanding and assert-ing their rights. Other aids include a free online resource from the Commission on Mental and Physical Disability Law at *www.abanet.org/disability/lawpract.htm*. You may also find other agencies in your state on the Bazelon Center website's list of state advocacy links at *www.bazelon.org/links/states/index.htm*.

Appendix E

USEFUL BOOKS AND RESOURCES

BOOKS ON ADHD

For Parents

Taking Charge of ADHD: The Complete, Authoritative Guide for Parents (revised edition)
Author: Russell A. Barkley
Publisher: Guilford Press, New York, NY, 2000, 321 pages

An outstanding resource for parents of children with attention deficit disorder with hyperactivity, *Taking Charge of ADHD* has now been revised and updated to incorporate the most current information on ADHD and its treatment. From internationally renowned ADHD expert Russell A. Barkley, the book empowers parents by arming them with up-to-date knowledge, expert guidance, and the confidence they need to ensure that their child receives the best care possible.

Give Your ADD Teen a Chance: A Guide for Parents of Teenagers with Attention Deficit Disorder
Author: Lynn Weiss
Publisher: Pinon Press, Colorado Springs, CO, 1996, 200 pages

This book provides parents with expert help by showing them how to determine which issues are caused by "normal" teenage development and which are caused by ADD. The book enables parents to look objectively at their ADD teen, giving guidelines for discipline, guidance, and responsibility.

For Kids and Teens

ADD/ADHD Behavior-Change Resource Kit: Ready-to-Use Strategies and Activities for Helping Children with Attention Deficit Disorder
Author: Grad L. Flick
Publisher: Jossey-Bass, San Francisco, 2002, 416 pages

(Books are listed alphabetically by first author's last name within each subsection.)

Virtually all you need to help kids take charge of their own behavior and build effective life and social skills, this book covers topics such as changing behaviors, building social skills, solving homework issues, and improving classroom behavior. The author details a proven set of training exercises and programs in which teachers, counselors, and parents work together to monitor and manage the child's behavior to achieve the desired results.

Learning to Slow Down and Pay Attention: A Book for Kids about ADD
Authors: Kathleen G. Nadeau, Ellen B. Dixon, and John Rose (Illustrator)
Publisher: Magination Press, Washington, DC, 1997, 80 pages
This workbook gives kids with ADD information on matters such as how to clean a room quickly and easily and how to make sure they do their homework on time. It is a fun-filled approach to learning how to get along better at school, with friends, and in life. The book is packed with cartoons, games, and activities. For parents, the book includes information on behavior management and on support groups.

A Bird's-Eye View of Life with ADD and ADHD: Advice from Young Survivors
Authors: Chris A. Zeigler Dendy and Alex Zeigler
Publisher: Cherish the Children, Cedar Bluff, AL, 2003, 180 pages
This book is a treasured resource for teenagers that gives first-hand advice from their peers. It was written by twelve teens and a young adult who are living with ADHD. In addition to factual information and practical strategies, this book gives teens and families a sense of hope that they too will survive this sometimes overwhelming disorder.

For Teachers

Teaching Teens with ADD and ADHD: A Quick Reference Guide for Teachers and Parents
Author: Chris A. Zeigler Dendy
Publisher: Woodbine House, Bethesda, MD, 2000, 352 pages
This book contains everything a teacher needs to know about ADHD in teens. *Teaching Teens with ADD and ADHD* contains concise summaries of over fifty key issues related to attention-deficit disorders and school success. Topics range from understanding the basics of ADHD to using effective interventions.

For All

Understanding ADHD: The Definitive Guide to Attention-Deficit/Hyperactivity Disorder
Authors: Kit Chee and Christopher Green
Publisher: Ballantine Books, New York, 1998, 336 pages
An invaluable resource for parents, teachers, and health professionals for informative, reassuring, and up-to-date information on ADHD. As renowned pediatrician Christopher Green explains, this disorder is actually a cluster of behaviors, including

inattentiveness, impulsiveness, and overactivity, that causes children to underachieve at school and behave poorly at home despite high intelligence and quality parenting.

Driven to Distraction: Recognizing and Coping with Attention Deficit Disorder from Childhood Through Adulthood
Authors: Edward M. Hallowell and John J. Ratey
Publisher: Touchstone Books, Carmichael, CA, 1995, 336 pages
This clear and valuable book dispels a variety of myths about attention deficit disorder. The authors attack the most two specific myths: that ADD is an issue only for children and that ADD relates simply to limited intelligence or limited self-discipline. The authors blatantly attack these myths by their own personal lives: both authors have ADD themselves and both are successful medical professionals. They cite Mozart and Einstein as examples of possible ADD sufferers. Although they warn against over-diagnosis, they also do a convincing job of answering the criticism that "everybody and therefore nobody" has ADD. Especially helpful are the lists of tips for dealing with ADD in a child, a partner, or a family member.

Attention Deficit Hyperactivity Disorder: State of the Science, Best Practices
Editors: Peter Jensen and James Cooper
Publisher: Civic Research Institute, Kingston, NJ, 2002, 686 pages
Written by researchers in the field of children's mental health, this book details the current best practices for ADHD. It is an in-depth guide to ADHD diagnosis, causes, treatment, and outcomes. Topics covered include biological bases and cognitive correlates of ADHD; controversies regarding over- and underdiagnosis of ADHD; risks and rewards of treatment with stimulant medication; the impact on individuals, families, and society; and much more. This book encompasses an overall view of the state of the science of ADHD. Available at *www.civicresearchinstitute.com*

ADHD Handbook for Families: A Guide to Communicating with Professionals
Author: Paul L. Weingartner
Publisher: Child Welfare League of America, Washington, DC, 1999, 146 pages.
This book is packed with proven, real-life strategies and techniques that can be put to use immediately. The *ADHD Handbook* is an excellent resource for anyone who wants to understand what ADHD is, what it feels like, and how to help children live a full life.

BOOKS ON MEDICATION

Medications for School-Age Children: Effects on Learning and Behavior
Authors: Ronald T. Brown and Michael G. Sawyer
Publisher: Guilford Press, New York, 1998, 228 pages
This book covers a broad array of issues from basic principles of pharmacological treatment to its social and cultural implications. It is a well-researched manual that provides a clear and concise account of the behavioral, affective, cognitive, and physiological changes associated with the use of psychotropic medication in children.

*Helping Parents, Youth, and Teachers Understand Medications for Behavioral and
    Emotional Problems: A Resource Book of Medication Information Handouts*
Editors: Mina K. Dulcan and Tami Benton
Publisher: American Psychiatric Press, Washington, DC, 2002, 202 pages
    Developed by experts at Children's Memorial Hospital in Chicago, this book is a
collection of handouts that cover today's most effective medications for pediatric
behavioral and emotional disorders, including anticonvulsants, stimulants, antianxiety
medications, and SSRIs.

*Pocket Guide for the Textbook of Pharmacotherapy for Child and Adolescent
    Psychiatric Disorders*
Authors: John Holttum and Samuel Gershon; editor: David Rosenberg
Publisher: Brunner-Routledge, New York, 1994, 555 pages
    This is a quick-reference guide for psychiatrists, therapists, social workers, and other
practitioners about each group of medications. It is a comprehensive textbook that focuses
on diagnostic issues relevant to dispensing psychotropic medications to children and adolescents, highlighting similarities and differences in treating children versus adults.

Stimulant Drugs and ADHD: Basic and Clinical Neuroscience
Editors: Mary V. Solanto, Amy F. T. Arnsten, and F. Xavier Castellanos
Publisher: Oxford University Press, Oxford, UK, 2001, 410 pages
    This technical book illustrates a comprehensive description of the clinical features
of ADHD and the clinical response to stimulants. In addition, it details the neuroanatomy and functional neurophysiology of dopamine and norepinephrine systems
with respect to regulation of certain processes: arousal, activity, and impulse control.

Straight Talk about Psychiatric Medications for Kids (revised edition)
Author: Timothy E. Wilens
Publisher: Guilford Press, New York, 2004, 310 pages
    This essential book provides up-to-date information that enables readers to fully
understand what their child's doctor is recommending and what their options are. Har-
vard University researcher and practitioner Dr. Timothy Wilens explains which medications may be prescribed for children and why; examines effects on children's health,
emotions, and school performance; and helps parents become active, informed managers of their children's care.

BOOKS ON BEHAVIORAL THERAPY

*Cognitive-Behavioral Therapy with ADHD Children: Child, Family, and
    School Interventions*
Author: Lauren Braswell
Publisher: Guilford Press, New York, 1991, 391 pages
    This book overviews the status of ADHD and related conditions. The author suggests
practical guidelines for clinicians. The book's approach emphasizes the importance of the
active involvement of parents and school personnel in the child's treatment.

Cognitive and Behavioral Interventions: An Empirical Approach to Mental Health Problems
Authors: Linda W. Craighead, W. Edward Craighead, Alan E. Kazdin, and Michael J. Mahoney
Publisher: Pearson Allyn & Bacon, Upper Saddle River, NJ, 1993, 464 pages
This book covers disorders and problem areas in both adult and child/adolescent populations, reflects the views and conclusions of the active researchers in the field, and focuses on empirical validation and differing approaches in and across problem areas.

Promoting Health and Mental Health in Children, Youth, and Families
Author: David S. Glenwick; editor: Leonard A. Jason
Publisher: Springer, New York, 1993, 264 pages
Part of the Springer Series on Behavior Therapy and Behavioral Medicine, this book describes research on preventing specific physical, social, or mental health problems such as drug or sexual abuse, AIDS, and teenage pregnancy on a community basis through behavioral therapy.

You Mean I'm Not Lazy, Stupid or Crazy?!: A Self-Help Book for Adults with Attention Deficit Disorder
Authors: Kate Kelly, Peggy Ramundo, and Larry B. Silver
Publisher: Scribner, Princeton, NJ, 1996, 464 pages
This book contains straightforward, practical advice for taking control of the symptoms, minimizing the disabilities, and maximizing the advantages of adult ADD.

ADHD Book: Living Right Now!
Author: Martin L. Kutscher
Publisher: Greenleaf, Chagrin Falls, OH, 2003, 128 pages
The book focuses on overreactions, impulse control, easy frustration, time management, and organizational problems as key aspects of ADHD. It includes suggestions of how to overcome these organizational problems.

ADD and the College Student: A Guide for High School and College Students with Attention Deficit Disorder
Editor: Patricia O. Quinn
Publisher: Magination, Washington, DC, 1994, 128 pages
This concise handbook is packed with practical information and advice for the smoothest possible transition to college life, including lifestyle habits for a student's success.

The ADHD Book of Lists: A Practical Guide for Helping Children and Teens with Attention Deficit Disorders
Author: Sandra F. Rief
Publisher: Jossey-Bass, San Francisco, 2003, 320 pages
A comprehensive, reliable source of answers, practical strategies, and tools written in a convenient list format. It is filled with the strategies, supports, and interventions

that have been found to be the most effective in minimizing the problems and optimizing the success of children and teens with ADHD.

Think Good—Feel Good: A Cognitive Behavior Therapy Workbook for Children
Author: Paul Stallard
Publisher: Halsted Press, New York, 2002, 186 pages
   This book is an exciting and pioneering new practical resource for undertaking cognitive behavior therapy with children and young people. The materials have been developed by the author and tested extensively in clinical work with children and young people with a range of psychological problems.

The Organized Parent: 365 Simple Solutions to Managing Your Home, Your Time, and Your Family's Life
Author: Christina Tinglof
Publisher: McGraw Hill, New York, 2002, 256 pages
   This book contains a collection of tips and advice on how you can create an organized and efficient home and family schedule.

Treating Anger, Anxiety, and Depression in Children and Adolescents: A Cognitive-Behavioral Perspective
Author: Jerry Wilde
Publisher: Accelerated Development, London, 1996, 185 pages
   This is a guide to treating the most prevalent problems facing children and adolescents today, using rational-emotive behavior therapy. The author applies a cognitive-behavioral perspective in individual, group, school, or private settings.

Cognitive-Behavioral Assessment and Therapy with Adolescents
Author: Janet M. Zarb
Publisher: Brunner-Routledge, New York, 1992, 272 pages
   This book provides a general resource for various mental health professionals by offering a perspective that encompasses both the distinct set of behavioral, motivational, and cognitive features presented by the adolescent client and the overall social system in which the client lives.

RESOURCES ON ORGANIZATION/HOME AND TIME MANAGEMENT

Organization and time management present challenges for many people, but can be especially challenging for individuals with ADHD. The hallmark traits of ADHD, inattention and distractibility, make organization and management of time and money very difficult, requiring the individual to implement various structures and processes and to utilize tools such as day planners and reminders. The following web site, "Time Management: Learning to Use a Day Planner—A Guide to Organizing the Home and Office," offers more information on time management and on use of a day planner:
   www.help4adhd.org/organization.cfm

Other Helpful Tips for Organization Skills:

- Use to-do lists and day planners
- Use timers and alarms, either through a clock, watch, PDA, or computer
- Attend to daily tasks, such as filing documents or paying bills
- Color-code file folders, textbooks, and binders
- Designate specific areas for easily misplaced items such as keys and bills
- Break down large projects into smaller, manageable steps

Eichermuller, P. (2002). (article) *Taking control of your clutter.* (*www.sunshineorganizing.com*).

Gracia, M. (2002). *www.getorganizednow.com* (forum).

Hall, J. (2002). *www.overhall.com.*

Kolberg, J., & Nadeau, K. (2002). *ADD-friendly ways to organize your life.* New York: Brunner-Routledge.

Moulding, C. (2002). Ten ideas for quick clutter control. *Get Organized Now Newsletter.* (*www.getorganizednow.com*).

Schechter, H. (2001). *Let go of clutter.* New York: McGraw-Hill (*www.letgoclutter.com*).

Winston, S. (1995). *Stephanie Winston's best organizing tips.* New York: Simon & Schuster.

Morgenstern, J. (1998). *Organizing from the inside out.* New York: Henry Holt.

BLANK ACTION PLANS

SHORT-TERM ACTION PLAN

Your child's needs	Approaches How will the need(s) be addressed? Resources?	Who will do it? Who else will assist and be on your child's team?	When? What is the time frame for accomplishing specific tasks?	Outcomes Short-term goals and objectives
Social–emotional needs				
Medical needs				
Educational needs				
Parent–family needs				

INTERMEDIATE-TERM ACTION PLAN

Your child's needs	Approaches How will the need(s) be addressed? Resources?	Who will do it? Who else will assist and be on your child's team?	When? What is the time frame for accomplishing specific tasks?	Outcomes Intermediate-term goals and objectives
Social–emotional needs				
Medical needs				
Educational needs				
Parent–family needs				

LONG-TERM ACTION PLAN

Your child's needs	Approaches How will the need(s) be addressed? Resources?	Who will do it? Who else will assist and be on your child's team?	When? What is the time frame for accomplishing specific tasks?	Outcomes Long-term goals and objectives
Social–emotional needs				
Medical needs				
Educational needs				
Parent–family needs				

Appendix G

TABLE OF PSYCHIATRIC DISORDERS, SYMPTOMS, AND PROVEN TREATMENTS

Diagnosis	Symptoms	Scientifically proven treatments

Disruptive Behavior Disorders

Diagnosis	Symptoms	Scientifically proven treatments
Attention-deficit/hyperactivity disorder (ADHD)	• Inattention, impulsivity, and hyperactivity are three types of behaviors and indicators. • Becoming easily distracted, rarely following instructions, and losing and forgetting things are signs of inattention. • Fidgeting, squirming, blurting out answers, and having difficulty waiting in line or for a turn are signs of impulsivity and hyperactivity.	• *Behavior therapy.* • *A combination of medication,* specifically stimulants, *and behavior therapy* has been found to be the most effective treatment choice. • *Classroom accommodations.* • *Stimulants:* Concerta, Metadate, Focalin, Ritalin, Adderall, Dexedrine, and Cylert all reduce children's hyperactivity and improve their ability to focus, work, and learn. • *Other medications:* Stratterra, Wellbutrin, and some tricyclic antidepressants have been shown to be effective.
Conduct disorder (CD)	• Frequent temper tantrums, aggression towards people and/or animals, has violated the rights of others by stealing or engaging in vandalism. • Up to about 25% of children and up to 50% of adolescents with ADHD also have CD.	• Considered one of the most difficult diagnoses to treat, there is not one medication or therapy of choice. • Often a child with conduct disorder has another diagnosis (e.g., ADHD), so the therapist will begin treatment with a medication and/or therapy that is effective in reducing the symptoms of the other diagnosis. • *Medication* may be used to reduce the child's negative behavior. • *Behavior therapy,* depending on the age of the child, can be effective. • *Parent training and videotaped modeling of parent training* have also been found to be effective in helping parents in managing their child's behavior. *(cont.)*

Diagnosis	Symptoms	Scientifically proven treatments
Oppositional defiant disorder (ODD)	• Extreme levels of argumentativeness, disobedience, stubbornness, negativity, and aggravation of others are signs. ODD is a often a precursor to conduct disorder. • Up to about 40% of those with ADHD also have ODD.	• *Behavior therapy.* • Certain forms of *group therapy* that use behavioral therapy techniques have shown benefit.

Anxiety disorders

Diagnosis	Symptoms	Scientifically proven treatments
Generalized anxiety disorder	• Constant worrying about normal everyday activities. • Always expecting the worst when there is no reason to think this way. • Complaining of physical problems like headache, nausea, tiredness, or muscle ache. • Up to about 30% of children with ADHD also have anxiety disorders.	• *Cognitive-behavioral therapy* • Teaches the child to control both the behavior and thoughts in situations that cause anxiety. • Works best for older children and adolescents because it requires the child to talk about thoughts and feelings.
Obsessive–compulsive disorder	• Repeated, unwanted obsessive thoughts, for example, children may demand that things be done in a certain way or that questions be answered over and over again. • Compulsive behaviors that seem impossible to stop, like constantly washing hands, touching, counting, or checking things.	• *Selective serotonin reuptake inhibitors (SSRIs)* • A category of several medications; Prozac, Zoloft, Paxil, Celexa, and Luvox are SSRIs. • Zoloft, Paxil, and Luvox are the only SSRIs that have been approved by the Food and Drug Administration (FDA) for use in children. Paxil's use is somewhat controversial because of the possibility that it might increase the risk of suicidal thinking or behavior in depressed youth. • *Cognitive-behavioral therapy* is being tested.
Panic disorder	• Repeated occurrences of intense fear that happen often and without warning. • Physical signs of a panic attack include chest pain, heart palpitations, shortness of breath, dizziness, and stomach pain.	• *Cognitive-behavioral therapy*

Diagnosis	Symptoms	Scientifically proven treatments
Specific phobia	• Extreme fear of something that has little or no actual danger that leads to the avoidance of objects or situations. • Crying, tantrums, freezing, or clinging are associated behaviors.	• *Behavioral therapy* • Focuses on figuring out ways for the child to change his or her behavior by using a goal-oriented system, often with small rewards. • Positive and negative reinforcement is usually an important part of the therapy. • A reward system may be set up that includes mild punishments, such as the loss of certain privileges to help motivate the child to change his or her behavior.
Posttraumatic stress disorder	• After experiencing a traumatic event such as child abuse, rape, or natural disasters, the child experiences recurring nightmares, flashbacks, emotional numbness, depression, or anger. • Irritability and being easily startled are indicators.	• *Cognitive-behavioral therapy*

Mood Disorders

Diagnosis	Symptoms	Scientifically proven treatments
Major depression	• Feelings of hopelessness, helplessness, worthlessness, inability to concentrate, irritability, change in appetite, change in sleep pattern, and loss of energy are signs. • Ten to thirty percent of those with ADHD also have depression.	• *Interpersonal therapy* • A short form of psychotherapy in which the child evaluates his or her own interaction with others. • Emphasis is placed on the child's current social development by focusing on any self-imposed isolation. • *Cognitive-behavioral therapy* and *SSRIs* have also been found to be effective. • Only Prozac has been approved by the FDA for the treatment of depression in youth.
Dysthymia	• A milder, more chronic form of depression. Only the lows are experienced and rarely the highs. The child does not attach pleasure to things that should make him or her happy.	• *Cognitive-behavioral therapy, SSRIs*

(cont.)

Diagnosis	Symptoms	Scientifically proven treatments
Bipolar disorder	• Extreme mood swings from high to low. The high state is called *mania* or *hypomania* and is characterized by rapid speech, impulsive or reckless behavior, irritability, and racing thought processes. • In the low state, *depression,* the child experiences difficulty concentrating, difficulty sleeping, changes in appetite, decreased energy, and a feeling of hopelessness. • Up to twenty percent of those with ADHD also have bipolar disorder. (This high percentage reflects the finding that although ADHD symptoms are often seen first, bipolar disorder is usually the primary or underlying disorder.)	• Treatments have not yet been well tested for use in children and adolescents. • To date we know that a combination of treatment methods results in the best outcome for children. • *Psychotherapy and psychoeducation* • Involves talking between the child and therapist to bring about change in the child's behavior in managing the condition. • Educating the child and family on warning signs of mania and managing the episodes. • *Medication* • Lithium has been found to be effective in treating manic and depressive symptoms. • Depakote and Tegretol have been found to be effective for young adults and may be useful for children. • Other medications may have a role in treatment for children and adolescents.

Disorders Usually First Diagnosed in Infancy, Childhood, or Adolescence

Autism	• Delay in or total lack of development of communication skills. May repeat words or phrases, misuse pronouns, or invent new words. • Difficulty in social interactions. • Restricted range of activities or interests. • Disturbances in the use of nonverbal behaviors, such as eye-to-eye gaze, facial expressions, body postures, and gestures. • Little or no interest in making friends or social play. • Stereotypical behavior (hand flapping, body rocking).	• Treatment programs that produce the greatest gains involve parents, build on the child's interests, offer a predictable schedule, teach tasks as a series of simple steps, actively engage the child's attention in highly structured activities, and provide regular reinforcement of behavior. • No medication can yet correct the brain structures or impaired nerve connections that seem to underlie autism. However, some medications (such as Risperdal and haloperidal) have been found to be effective in reducing the child's behaviors that make it hard to function. • Very intensive behavioral therapy has been helpful in decreasing negative behaviors and, for some children, has returned them to more normal functioning.

Diagnosis	Symptoms	Scientifically proven treatments
Asperger's syndrome	• Extreme difficulty in social interactions. • Repetitive and restricted patterns of behavior, interests, and activities such as movements with hands, fingers, or whole-body. • No delay in the development of language.	• Depending on the severity of the child's symptoms and behaviors, combinations of treatment methods that involve individual and family therapy and medication are often used. There is little evidence to show that any one treatment is better than another.
Learning disorders (LDs)	• Significantly lower than expected achievement on a reading, math, or writing standardized test given a child's age, schooling, and level of intelligence. • Up to about twenty-five percent of those with ADHD also have LDs.	• Treatment usually focuses on helping the child learn new ways to process and understand materials. Sometimes special accommodations are needed in the classroom (e.g., extra time for test taking, computers to help with writing, etc.).
Communication disorders	• Difficulty understanding or producing language. • Stuttering.	• *Speech and language therapy*
Tics and Tourette syndrome	• Facial tics and motor tics like head jerking or foot stamping. • Uttering strange or unacceptable sounds, words, or phrases. • Touching people excessively and repeatedly. • Rare cases of shouting obscenities. • Fewer than seven percent of those with ADHD also have tics or Tourette syndrome.	• Often no medication or treatment is needed if the tics do not interfere with functioning. • If tics begin to interfere with functioning, medications such as clonidine, haloperidol, pimozide, fluphenazine, and clonazepam can be used. • Although not a psychological problem, psychotherapy may be beneficial to the patient in dealing with the social and emotional aspects of the disorder.
Adjustment disorder	• Results from an identifiable stressor such as a transitional period (divorce), interpersonal problem, or crisis. • Affective (emotional) or behavioral symptoms. • Distress. • Impairment in functioning.	• Most adjustment disorder symptoms disappear on their own with removal of the stressor (within six months). • If symptoms persist longer than six months, a full evaluation should be done to identify any other disorders that may be present.
Aggressive and reckless behavior (harmful to self and others)	• Severe aggressive thoughts expressed about others or self. • Severe aggressive or harmful acts geared toward injuring others or self. • Reckless behavior without regard for dangerous consequences.	• Always insure the safety of the child or others in danger first, seeking immediate help if necessary (police, ambulance, etc.). • Once child is stabilized, seek additional professional help in order to identify causes of dangerous behavior and treat the symptoms.

Appendix H

SAMPLE LETTERS

Appeal Letter to an Insurance Company for Turning Down a Claim

Healthcare Plan
ATTN: Mrs. My Phone Contact within the Company
Address
City, State, Zip

Dear _____:

I am writing with respect to your company's denial of my claim for my out-of-pocket expenses for my son Robert's medication needed for treatment of his severe Attention-Deficit/Hyperactivity Disorder (314.01), a medical condition that often results in severe long-term impairment and life-long morbidity.

I wish to formally appeal this decision, on the following grounds:

First, Dr. Verywell Qualified has provided treatment for the last three years, ever since Robert was first diagnosed. Despite Dr. Qualified's substantial treatment expertise in this area, no medications proved effective and tolerable in terms of side-effects, until Dr. Qualified tried Robert on NewDrug four months ago. This new treatment has made an enormous difference in Robert's life, and for the first time in years he is looking forward to school, and getting good grades as well.

Unfortunately, I was informed that this medication is "not covered" because it is slightly more expensive that some of the older forms of medication, and my two previous claims submitted for reimbursement were denied (see attached). Because I could not afford to continuing paying these without the insurance copayment, I was forced to have Robert put back on OldMed last month, and it has been a disaster. OldMed was the most effective of all of the previous medications tried, but basically, it DOES NOT WORK for my son. I understand the need to keep costs down by encouraging plan subscribers to use the most economical forms of treatment whenever possible. However, this has been tried, and my son is now suffering considerably since he has had to go back on the much less effective medication he was on before.

Dr. Verywell Qualified has written a letter attesting to Robert's need for this particular form of medication, and the inadequacy of earlier treatments tried, including the ones covered in the current healthcare plan.

Please contact me at your earliest convenience concerning the outcome of this appeal.

Sincerely,

Parent

cc: My Employer's Benefits Manager (Personnel/Human Resources Department)
My State's Insurance Commissioner
Dr. Verywell Qualified

Enclosures: Claims for reimbursement, dated dd/mm/yyyy and dd/mm/yyyy

Letter to Your Principal Requesting an Evaluation
for an IEP or a 504 Plan

Principal
Local School
Address
City, State, Zip

Dear _____:

I would like to request an evaluation of my son Robert [full name and student ID# or date of birth] for his eligibility for special education provisions (IDEA) and/or Section 504 accommodations. I have been concerned that he/she is not progressing well in school and that he/she may need some special help in order to learn. He/she is in the [grade level and name of current teacher].

For the last two years both of his classroom teachers have noted that he has substantial problems completing assignments, problems with excessive motor behavior, and impulsivity. Please note that Dr. Verywell Qualified has recently evaluated and diagnosed my son as having Attention-Deficit/Hyperactivity Disorder. Because Dr. Verywell Qualified was concerned that Robert's ADHD was resulting in decreased alertness and impairment in school performance and learning, he requested us to pursue these school-based evaluations, in order to get my son the help he needs.

I understand that the evaluation is to be provided at no charge to me. My reasons for requesting this procedure are ... [keep this paragraph short, but give one or two reasons for your concern about your child].

I would appreciate meeting with each person who will be doing the evaluation before he/she tests my child so that I might share information about (child's name) with him/her. I will also expect a copy of the written report generated by each evaluator so that I might review it before the IEP [or 504 Plan] meeting.

It is my understanding that I have to provide written permission for these tests to be administered and I will be happy to do so upon receipt of the proper forms and explanation of the process.

Please contact me at your earliest convenience so that we may begin the next steps in planning for an evaluation.

Sincerely,

Parent

[*Note*: Remember to send this letter by certified mail or hand deliver it. If you hand deliver it, have the school official sign and date a receipt so that you will have documentation of it. Remember also to keep a copy for your file.]

Used with permission of Mary Durheim.

Appeal Letter to Your School District for Unacceptable IDEA or Section 504 Recommendations
(Sample Letter Requesting a Due Process Hearing)

Assistant Superintendent
Special Education Programs
School District Headquarters
Address
City, State, Zip

Dear _____:

I would like to request a due process hearing under the procedures and protections outlined in _____ [specify either IDEA or Section 504]. Please note that my son Robert was evaluated for special education placement on Day, Month, Year, and an Individual Education Plan was developed that I feel is not appropriate for addressing my child's special education needs.

   We have tried to resolve the issue(s) of: _____

_____

[List the specific issue(s) of concern. Be brief but specific.]

   We are willing to meet with you and the hearing officer in a pre-hearing conference. We would like a list of any free or low-cost legal advocacy help available in this area plus a copy of our due process rights under _____ [specify either Section 504 or the IDEA].

   We regret that we have had to come to this method of resolution but feel it is necessary. We expect to hear from you soon.

                              Sincerely,

                              Parent

cc: My Lawyer, Esq.
    State Department of Education

Enclosures: IEP [or 504 Plan] for Robert Roberts, dated dd/mm/yyyy

[*Note*: Be sure to send this certified with return receipt requested to insure compliance with any timelines that may be applicable. Remember to keep a copy of this letter for your file and indicate anyone else to whom you are sending copies by "cc" at bottom of letter.]

Used with permission of Mary Durheim

Letter Requesting Records (for IDEA or Section 504)

For IDEA, use <u>underlined</u> words, for 504, use words in parentheses ( ).

Date:

To: <u>Special Education Director</u> (Section 504 Coordinator) and/or Principal
         School District
         Address

From:

I am the parent of _____, DOB: _____
        I am requesting a copy of any and all educational records held in any form and
in any location by _____ School District. This re-
quest is made pursuant to 34 CFR §104.36 and §99.7 (FERPA). My child's educational records should include (but is not limited to) the following: all reports written as
a result of the school's evaluation; reports of independent evaluators; medical/health
records; discipline reports and/or any disciplinary hearings and decisions; atten-
dance records and/or any truancy records; summary reports of <u>special education</u>
(504) committee meetings with attached minutes; any <u>special education</u> (504) eligibility committee meetings; my child's <u>Individualized Education Plan</u> (Individual Accommodations Plan); and any correspondence between school officials, teachers, and myself.
        I understand that someone will be available to answer any questions I may have
regarding my son's/daughter's school records.
        I look forward to meeting with you in the near future. Please advise as to when
you will have the above requested information available and what, if any, charge
for reproduction you anticipate. If you have any questions, please call me at
_____.

_____
Signature of Parent

_____
Date Received

_____
Signature of School Personnel Receiving Request

[*Note*: Take this letter to the person listed above or send by certified mail. Have them
sign that they received this request. Make sure to keep a signed copy for your records.]

_____

Appeal Letter to Your School District about How a Section 504 Plan Is Being Implemented or When Insufficient Help Is Given to Assist Your Child

Assistant Superintendent
Section 504 Programs
School District Headquarters
Address
City, State, Zip

Dear _____:

Under the procedures and protections outlined under the Section 504 of the Civil Rights Code the Rehabilitation Act of 1973, I would like to inform you officially that despite my repeated verbal requests and discussions with school personnel, including Principal Well-Intended and Teacher CaresVeryMuch, the accommodations offered in my child's 504 Plan are not being implemented as agreed upon. The original 504 Plan, dated dd/mm/yyyy, is enclosed.

I should note that my child has been also independently evaluated by Dr. Verywell Qualified. After a comprehensive diagnostic evaluation, Dr. Qualified diagnosed Robert with severe Attention-Deficit/Hyperactivity Disorder, and verified that his ADHD is resulting in severely decreased alertness in academic tasks as well as impairment in school performance and learning. In addition, Dr. Qualified made specific recommendations concerning the types of provisions that Robert will need, if he is to be assured of a free and appropriate education and assured of his rights. As you will see by comparing Dr. Qualified's evaluation with the actual 504 Plan that was written (both are enclosed), the 504 Plan provisions fall far short of what Dr. Qualified determined is required.

Please contact me at your earliest convenience so that we can find a way to more satisfactorily ensure that Robert's rights under Section 504 of the Civil Rights Code of the Rehabilitation Act of 1973 are fully met. I will look forward to hearing from you.

Sincerely,

Parent

cc: My Lawyer, Esq.
    State Department of Education

Enclosures:
    Section 504 Plan for Robert Roberts, dated dd/mm/yyyy
    Medical Report/Evaluation from Dr. Verywell Qualified

Letter from Your Child's Doctor to Your School Concerning Your Child's Need for Special Assistance

Principal
Tom Dooley Elementary School

Attention: Special Education Team
County Public Schools

James Madison is the six-year-old son of Mark and Molly Madison. James was first seen by me in December 2002, at age 4, due to significant problems with opposition-ality and hyperactivity. Since that time, James has received medical treatment from me, as well as intensive behavior therapy from Gilbert GoodGuy, PhD.

Despite these intensive medical efforts, James has significant continuing difficulties in home and school functioning. Now in first grade, he remains very sensitive, easily provoked, and often needs intensive one-on-one support and supervision, such as is only available in a self-contained classroom. Without close supervision and availabil-ity of trained teachers who can work with children with SED (Serious Emotional Distur-bance), James's anxieties escalate, and he is prone to aggressive outbursts and/or so-cial withdrawal. Based on my evaluation, James's current diagnoses are the following:

1. Attention-Deficit/Hyperactivity Disorder
2. Oppositional Defiant Disorder
3. Anxiety Disorder, Not Otherwise Specified

School Recommendations: In addition to ongoing pharmacological management and home-based behavioral therapy, it is my professional opinion that James will need ad-ditional school-based interventions, to include the following:

1. Close coordination between home and school in giving home-based behavioral rewards.
2. A self-contained classroom where he can have the necessary assistance of an aide and SED-trained teachers with a 1:6 teacher–pupil ratio.
3. Monitoring for medication effects.

Under the guidelines of the Individuals with Disabilities Education Act (IDEA), PL 101-476, I recommend that James receive full psychological and educational evaluations to determine/confirm the presence of a disability, which can then be reviewed at an Special Education Team meeting for consideration of special educational resources and an Individualized Educational Plan (IEP) to assist James is achieving appropriate benefit from the school's educational program. I shall be glad to consult with and an-swer questions for the IEP team by conference call.

Thank you for your attention to this matter. Please do not hesitate to contact me if you have any questions in this regard.

Sincerely,

Verywell Qualified, MD

Appendix I

USING BEHAVIORAL STRATEGIES TO HELP YOUR CHILD IMPROVE HIS OR HER BEHAVIOR

Focus on the positive.
- List at least three good things about your child. Your child has wonderful qualities and strengths; it is important to remind yourself of these.
- List at least three good things about how you parent your child.
- Post these lists on your refrigerator.
- Celebrate them!

Try to redirect (not stop) troublesome behaviors.
- Children with ADHD are energetic, spontaneous, and have a short attention span (there's so much to do!). Reminders in a neutral tone, such as "Remember, we're getting ready for school," can be all a child needs to stay on task. It will also take less of your energy.

Create a consistent set of rewards that your child can earn by good behavior.
- **Start small**. Pick one or two behaviors to start with; for example, decreasing temper outbursts or talking back.
- **Keep expectations simple**. For example, when asked to clean his or her room or take his or her plates to the sink, the expectation is that your child will not argue, cry, shout, or some other undesirable response.
- **Motivate your child** by making a **chart** of his or her behavior.
- **Use stickers or stars (tokens)** to represent successful behavior. For example, if your child takes his or her plate to the sink without difficulty, he or she earns a star that is placed on the chart.
- **Your child receives a reward**, such as a small toy, a trip to the movies, or special time with a parent, after he or she earns a certain number of stars or tokens.
- **Make earning stars within your child's reach**. Behavior management through systems of reward work only when the child is able to see the consequences of good behavior. Set expectations that you know your child can meet, even if it falls short of the behavior you are trying to improve.

- **Younger children need more immediate rewards**. A week may be too long to associate good behavior with a reward. Try finding a reward that can be earned by a fewer number of stars. Try a reward such as "extra TV time" or "extra time on the computer" that can be rewarded in the same day.
- **Your child's behavior may get worse before it gets better**, as she or he "tests" how consistent the rules and consequences are.
- See the sample special reward charts on pages 270–271. For more assistance on using such methods, refer to Appendix E, Useful Books and Resources.

Providing structure is critical.
- Establishing consistent rules and schedules go a long way in helping your child manage tasks and activities.

Do not expect more than your child can manage.
- Avoid too much stimulation. Many people with ADHD have trouble screening out the many sights and sounds that most people can ignore. Noisy places or the colorful multiitem displays used in stores may be overstimulating for your child and may make it difficult to control his or her behavior.
- Choose child care that has a low child-to-adult ratio.
- Avoid formal gatherings, shopping trips, or eating out if these are more than your child can handle.

Plan ahead for difficult environments.
- Set up a special reward or privilege for obeying established rules and behaving properly during an outing or event.
- Review rules and punishment (loss of privileges) prior to the event/outing.

Prepare for transitions.
- Review the day's events in advance to help give an idea of what's going to happen.
- Give warnings 15, 10, and 5 minutes prior to a shift in activities or departure.

Routine, routine, routine!
- Meals, toileting, chores, and bedtime should be as regular as you can make them.

Catch 'em being good!
- Positive comments should outnumber negative comments by at least 2 to 1; work toward 5 to 1.
- Tell your child what you like to see and comment when he or she does it. For example, "I liked the way you waited your turn to use the bike. You did a **super** job!"
- Ignore harmless negative behavior (annoying noises, repeated questions, etc.).

Let your child know what you want him or her to do.
- Say "walk, please" instead of "don't run."
- Give only one instruction at a time.
- Some children with ADHD have a hard time listening when they are trying to

do something else (i.e., tying shoes). Give your child important information when he or she can listen.

- Have a formal program of positive reinforcement in place at both home and school—use tokens, stickers, even candies.

Establish consistent discipline.

- Less is more—make a few clear rules and consistently enforce them.
- Act quickly—talk (and threaten) less.
- Use nonphysical punishment—brief time-outs (young children) or loss of privileges (older children).

Stretch his or her attention span.

- Reward nonhyperactive behavior with praise, thumbs up, or a hug.
- Limit play materials available at one time but change them often.

Communicate frequently with your child's teacher.

- Work together to make rules and consequences consistent.
- Speak up for your child.
- Teach teachers, family, and friends about ADHD.

Give children frequent, positive feedback.

- Break activities into small steps.
- Create lists of steps to guide longer tasks.

Provide a safe place for free play!

Sample Chart for a School-Age Child

ROBIN'S SPECIAL REWARDS CHART

Morning routine—Week of Nov. 12–16

Item	Reward
*Get out of bed after 2 requests	2 Tickets
*Put on your clothes that are laid out	2 Tickets
*Brush teeth	2 Tickets
*Come to breakfast after 2 requests	1 Tickets
*Take your backpack to school with you	2 Tickets
*Go out and wait for the school bus by 8:15 A.M.	3 Tickets
TOTAL that can be earned daily	12 Tickets

	Monday	Tuesday	Wednesday	Thursday	Friday	Weekly total
Daily totals						

What I can purchase with my TICKETS

1. ½ hour TV time in the evening on school days	3 Tickets
2. Ice cream cone	3 Tickets
3. ½ hour of Daddy's time to help me with my home work	3 Tickets
4. 1 hour of computer games	5 Tickets
5. A toy valued at $10.00	25 Tickets

Instructions:

1. Set up the plan based on the desired change.
2. Determine the reward or payout (in this case we are using raffle tickets).
3. Keep the plan simple.
4. Determine the payout section with the child, based on rewards that will motivate him or her to earn the points/tickets.
5. Post the chart in an area of the home that is visible and can be checked often, generally the refrigerator.
6. Set up new chart each week.

Sample chart courtesy of Beth Kaplanek, RN.

Sample Chart for a Teen

Roger—Basic Allowance $10.00

Home

	Yes	No	10:00 P.M. lights out @ $1.00 per day
	Yes	No	
Sun.			
Mon.			
Tues.			
Weds.			
Thurs.			

School

			Assignments recorded in planner @ $1.00 per day
	Yes	No	
Sun.			
Mon.			
Tues.			
Weds.			
Thurs.			

1. 90 on a test—$5.00
2. 85 on a test—$3.00
3. 82 average for 1 quarter—bonus!

Upcoming test in _____   Date _____

Upcoming test in _____   Date _____

Payday is Friday (morning)—Remind me!

Sample chart courtesy of Beth Kaplanek, RN.

WAYS TO BECOME INVOLVED

HOW TO PARTICIPATE IN RESEARCH

This webpage of the National Institute of Mental Health (*www.nimh.nih.gov/studies/ clinres.cfm*) details how you can become involved in research and what this research will entail. Without the participation of patients with mental illness and other volunteers, the advances of tomorrow will not be realized. Most people who agree to take part in studies of mental illness hope the research will produce knowledge about the disease itself—for example, the role of genetics in illness—or about treatments that will benefit them directly.

It is important to note that just as research on treatments has evolved and become more effective, so too has our society's attentiveness to the well-being of research volunteers grown. Procedures now in place to protect volunteers are more effective than ever before.

For more information on research into the brain, behavior, and mental disorders, contact:

National Institute of Mental Health (NIMH)
Office of Communication and Public Liaison
Information Resources and Inquiries Branch
6001 Executive Boulevard, Room 8184, MSC 9663
Bethesda, MD 20892-9663
301-443-4513 (tel)
301-443-4279 (fax)
nimhinfo@nih.gov (e-mail)

HOW TO BECOME AN ADVOCATE

This webpage of Children and Adults with Attention-Deficit/Hyperactivity Disorder (*www.chadd.org/webpage.cfm?cat_id=7&subcat_id=62*) details how you can start a local chapter in your area or join the existing one. The five main goals of CHADD are to:

1. Provide a forum for continuing education on ADHD for parents, professionals, and adults.
2. Be a community resource for information about ADHD.
3. Maintain a support network for parents and caregivers who have children with ADHD and for adults with ADHD.
4. Make the best educational experiences available to children with ADHD so that their specific difficulties will be recognized and appropriately managed within educational settings.
5. Promote and influence legislative activities at the national, state, and local levels.

To accomplish these objectives CHADD needs support in communities at the grassroots level to advocate, educate, inform, and support—from people like you!

The first step is to request an information packet that will provide an overview explaining the different types of groups and the structure and responsibilities for each group. This includes "Startup Steps to Follow," a guide that will walk you through the startup process. Once you receive the packet, review it and call CHADD if you have any questions. Contact LaToya Wright, Chapter Services Coordinator, at 301-306-7070, ext. 121, or e-mail *latoya_wright@chadd.org*.

INDEX

ABOUT THE AUTHOR

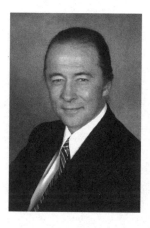

Peter S. Jensen, MD, is Director of the Center for the Advancement of Children's Mental Health—Putting Science to Work, and Ruane Professor of Child Psychiatry, both at the Columbia University College of Physicians and Surgeons in New York. Before coming to Columbia University, he was the Associate Director of Child and Adolescent Research at the National Institute of Mental Health (NIMH) in Bethesda, Maryland.

Dr. Jensen has written over two hundred articles and chapters for scientific and clinical journals, has edited or authored a dozen books on children's mental health research, and currently serves as coeditor or editorial board member of many journals. He has served on the Scientific Advisory Boards of the Tourette Syndrome Association, the Attention Deficit Disorder Association, and Children and Adults with Attention-Deficit/Hyperactivity Disorder (CHADD). He currently serves on the scientific advisory boards for the National Alliance for the Mentally Ill (NAMI) and the Medical Investigation of Neurologic Disorders (M.I.N.D.) Institute, as a member of the CHADD board of directors, and as the current president of the International Society of Research on Child and Adolescent Psychopathology. His research, writing, and teaching have been recognized by national awards from the major psychiatry, child psychiatry, psychology, and nursing associations, as well as NAMI and CHADD.

Dr. Jensen received his medical degree in 1978 from the George Washington University Medical School in Washington, DC. He did his postgraduate training at the University of California and at Letterman Army Medical Center, both in San Francisco. From there, he moved to NIMH, where he served as the lead NIMH investigator on the six-site NIMH- and U.S. Department of Education–funded Study of Multimodal Treatment of ADHD and worked on other multicenter studies.

Dr. Jensen's current areas of interest include the integration of research methods into clinical settings, effectiveness and dissemination research, and techniques for persuading medical practitioners and parents to adopt evidence-based mental health approaches in dealing with children who are suffering from mental disorders—"putting science to work."